Praise for *The Wellbeing Advantage*

The Wellbeing Advantage brilliantly connects the dots between movement, mindset, and meaningful change. A must-read for anyone who believes that sustainable wellbeing habits are the foundation of lifelong wellbeing.

Hugh Brasher,
CEO of London Marathon Events

The Wellbeing Advantage is an insightful read for anyone who wants to perform at a high level yet stay healthy and happy in the process. Dr Janine pushes you to honestly reflect on different aspects of your life, then offers concrete tips for building sustainable habits that work for YOU. To keep it doable, we are frequently reminded to approach change with flexibility and compassion. 'It's not about being perfect, but about being intentional.'

Each chapter includes practical tips for interpreting your wearable data in a meaningful way, without over-relying on it, followed by a section for those who get stressed by wearable data and prefer other means of learning. Even as someone who works with physiological data and sees a lot of value in it, I find this viewpoint very valuable! It lets the reader find themselves and the path that works for them.

The book made me revisit my own way of doing things and prompted me to add a few new habits into my routine – a very healthy exercise for all of us. Janine's approach to wellbeing is so comprehensive that I'm sure everyone will find something that will give them pause. A strong recommendation for individuals wanting to boost their wellbeing and performance as well as for coaches who work with high-performing clients.

Tiina Hoffman,
Exercise Physiologist and Master Trainer at Firstbeat Technologies

As a Lifestyle GP and triathlete, I see the same truth daily: small habits, repeated often, change health. *The Wellbeing Advantage* champions exactly that; simple, repeatable habits, plus smart use of wearable data that deliver the basics: sit less, move more, sleep better and feel it. Practical, evidence-based, and refreshingly free of fads.

Dr Hussain Al-Zubaidi, Lifestyle GP, TV Doctor,
RCGP Lifestyle & Physical Activity Champion

The Wellbeing Advantage offers busy professionals a comprehensive and practical guide to what thriving in the workplace and setting yourself up to be at your best requires. Dr Janine skilfully steers the reader through both stories and research to bust some myths and clear the way to build some new wellbeing habits.

Cath Bishop,
Olympian, Leadership & Culture Coach and
***Author of* The Long Win**

The Wellbeing Advantage is a timely, practical, and empowering guide for anyone seeking to thrive in today's demanding, modern world. Dr Janine van Someren distils cutting-edge, science-based insights, found at the unique intersection of elite performance coaching and HRV (heart rate variability) technology.

What truly makes this book stand out is its genuine compassion for the reader. Through many years of coaching teams and individuals, the author has clearly developed an empathetic and warm approach, which demonstrates a deep understanding of the everyday trials faced by her audience. Her method provides seven clear and actionable habits to live with greater purpose, energy, and resilience, without burning out.

Insightful, inspiring, and immediately useful, this is a must-read for anyone who wants to bring their best self to meet the opportunities and challenges of the modern world.

Adrian Kelly,
***Author of* The Success Complex**

As someone deeply committed to empowering others on their journey toward healing and self-awareness, I am delighted to endorse *The Wellbeing Advantage* by Dr Janine van Someren. I had the pleasure of speaking with Janine on my podcast in March 2023, where we explored how even the smallest changes can create profound shifts in our overall wellbeing. That powerful conversation left a lasting impression, and her book takes that message even further.

Janine's approach is refreshingly grounded and accessible. With compassion and clarity, she offers evidence-based habits that are simple to implement, yet deeply impactful for anyone navigating a busy life. *The Wellbeing Advantage* is more than just a guide – it's a supportive companion for anyone seeking sustainable energy, resilience, and long-term wellness without overwhelm.

Janine's wisdom is a gift to anyone ready to make positive, lasting change in their lives – one small, meaningful step at a time.

Sharon Fitzmaurice, Holistic Wellness Coach,
***Author and Host of* The Sharon Fitzmaurice Podcast**

'What gets measured gets managed', so they say… but only if you know how to respond. Otherwise, the constant stream of stats can quickly become overwhelming and, ironically, a source of anxiety in itself.

The Wellbeing Advantage is the handbook that should come with every wellness wearable. Written by Dr Janine van Someren – a distinguished wellness consultant, coach, and lecturer – this book helps readers make sense of the numbers their devices produce and shows them how to turn these insights into meaningful action.

Backed by research in physiology, neuroscience, positive psychology, and sports and behavioural science – and illustrated with compelling case studies from her coaching practice – Janine demonstrates how small, consistent, and sustainable habit shifts can give us a real advantage that supports not only our health and wellbeing, but our performance too.

The Wellbeing Advantage doesn't just unlock the meaning in the data, it shows us what to do with it, and how to move away from passive monitoring and into active self-leadership. So, enough with the sleep score navel-gazing – this book shows you how to actually do something about it.

Sophia Hodges,
Founder of Human Energy Optimisation

The Wellbeing Advantage is a wonderful tool to help anyone make long lasting changes in health, life, and performance. It aligns small steps in lifestyle pillars with wearable technology feedback and guides you to success. A great read and invaluable guide. I strongly recommend following all the steps in the order they are laid out.

Dr Robert Kelly, Cardiology MD MBA,
***Lifestyle Medicine Consultant, Heart Health Transformation Coach, and Author of* The Heart Book *and* Unlocking Success**

The Wellbeing Advantage is a clear, accessible, and genuinely useful read. Dr Janine van Someren has done a brilliant job of translating complex science, particularly around wearable tech, HRV, performance and stress, into practical strategies that are easy to understand and apply in a meaningful way.

It's a great resource for anyone who wants to perform optimally and stay well in a fast-paced world where chronic stress is unavoidable. I'll definitely be recommending it to my clients and adding it to the reading lists for my training resources. It's exactly the kind of evidence-based, practical guide we need more of in the wellbeing space.

Dr Bernadette Dancy,
Founder and Director of Stress Ed.

This is a brilliant book that cuts through the overwhelming noise around wellbeing, with complete clarity. In a space where advice can feel contradictory or unachievable, this book offers realistic techniques grounded in scientific research and evidence. The insights are accessible without ever being over-simplified and the practical steps focussed around seven themes of wellbeing are genuinely actionable. It offers strategies that easily integrate into daily life whatever your circumstances. What I particularly valued is the tone: it's supportive and authentic, never patronizing or prescriptive. This book is credible and trustworthy and a 'must-read' for every adult who's not sure where to start but wants to make a positive shift in their own wellness.

Lucy Clemas, CIPD Fellow,
Founder of The People Mix, People & Culture Strategist

As a former elite athlete, I've lived the realities of intense pressure, high expectations, and the constant pursuit of peak performance. *The Wellbeing Advantage* is a powerful toolkit for managing stress, sustaining energy, and staying grounded when the pressure is on. Dr Janine van Someren combines scientific insight with real-world empathy to offer a practical path to resilience – this book is essential reading for anyone serious about performing at their best, without burning out.

Andy Baddeley,
Olympic Finalist and CEO of The Running Channel

A brilliant contemporary book on health and wellbeing, connecting our love of data with the pursuit of self-improvement.

Structured around your day, *The Wellbeing Advantage* becomes your trusted companion, guiding you to make small, impactful changes with longevity in mind. I particularly love how Dr Janine encourages us to use wearable tech to spot health trends over time, and using *this* information to inform habit change, rather than obsessing over every real-time notification.

This book provides clarity on how to apply modern health science to your own individual circumstances, setting *The Wellbeing Advantage* apart from most other health books. My morning routine is already reaping the rewards of having read it.

Rachel Philpotts,
***Author of* The Burnout Bible**

The Wellbeing Advantage is an outstanding example of applied behavioural science made personal, practical, and deeply impactful. Grounded in robust psychological and physiological evidence, this book transforms abstract wellbeing concepts into accessible and actionable strategies that genuinely support lasting change. Dr Janine van Someren demonstrates a rare ability to translate complexity into clarity. Through her compassionate coaching voice, relatable case stories, and behaviourally sound frameworks like the 'Aha Model', readers are empowered to move from insight to action without overwhelm or perfectionism. Her guidance is underpinned by behavioural principles including habit formation, self-reflection, and reinforcement, ensuring that new practices are not just adopted, but sustained.

This is not a prescriptive wellness manual; it's a behaviourally intelligent toolkit for anyone seeking to navigate stress, build resilience, and improve wellbeing through small, science-backed shifts. Whether or not you use wearable tech, the reflective prompts, micro-habit suggestions, and thoughtfully layered behavioural cues make change feel not only possible, but personal.

This book will help many people make evidence-based changes to their lives and, perhaps more importantly, understand why those changes matter and how to stick with them.

Dr Heather McKee,
Behaviour Change Specialist and Habit Change Speaker

This is a standout guide to building evidence-based wellbeing. *The Wellbeing Advantage* offers practical, scientific, and data-backed strategies and frameworks for creating sustainable health habits in the midst of busy lives. Grounded in easily digestible science and delivered with clarity, Janine expertly brings these strategies to life through relatable case studies that resonate. Janine's passion for her work shines on every page, and she delivers each behavioural nudge with the empathy and insight born of her own lived experience, personally and professionally. This is a valuable resource for high performers ready to lead their lives with wellbeing as their strategic advantage.

Dr Kellie Rose,
Performance Scientist and Executive Women's Health Coach

Most employees don't need another lecture on 'self-care', they need something that works on a busy Tuesday. *The Wellbeing Advantage* delivers exactly that. Janine blends solid science with clear, practical steps that guide smarter choices in the moments that matter: when to push, when to pause, how to focus, and how to recover at the right times.

What I like most is the usability; micro-habits you can slot into your schedule, quick reads you can act on immediately, and a simple way to see what genuinely improves your energy and performance, without adding to your to-do list. If you want to feel better and work better, start here.

Dr Phillip Bell,
CEO of ART Health Solutions

Janine and *The Wellbeing Advantage* takes years of knowledge and experience breaking it down into easy to understand gems that will truly improve performance and from there, life! I have been lucky enough to work one on one with Janine and felt the benefits, now with this book, you've got it all in your own hands.

Clare McKenna, Health & Wellness Coach,
***Broadcaster and Author of* Would You Be Well?**

The Wellbeing Advantage is a smart guide for high performers to maximize their energy and resilience with seven science-backed strategies. Using wearable technology and looking at measurements like HRV to help you make lifelong changes that will positively impact you for many years to come. A great read for those looking to thrive no matter how busy you are.

Nicole Goode,
Clinical Director & Founder of Goode Health,
***Author of* Optimal You**

In elite sport, there is no shortage of data but the gold lies in finding the right insights and applying them at the right time. What Janine has achieved in *The Wellbeing Advantage* is a rare and valuable bridge between high-performance data, practical behavioural science, and real-world application. Whether you're an athlete, executive, or someone seeking to perform at your best without burning out, this book offers a clear path forward. A timely and important contribution to the future of sustainable performance.

Dr Brian Moore, CEO of Orreco, High Performance Sport Scientist

The Wellbeing Advantage is an informative and inspiring read for anyone wanting to benefit from using data-based awareness to create a change in their lifestyle and health. Because Janine is speaking from personal experience, as well as her professional expertise, it makes this book even more powerful.

***Louise Lloyd, Author of* Stress Hacking**

The Wellbeing Advantage cuts through wellness noise with calm precision. Dr Janine van Someren pairs real physiology with behaviour you can actually do, using wearable trends to decide when to push and when to recover, without becoming a slave to the score. Practical, compassionate, and refreshingly free of fluff.

Dr Steve Ingham, Director of Supporting Champions and Athlete Now, Performance Scientist and Speaker

Dr Janine van Someren

THE WELLBEING ADVANTAGE

7 transformative habits to thrive in work and life

First published in Great Britain by Practical Inspiration Publishing, 2026

ISBN 9781788608855 (paperback)
9781788608848 (hardback)
9781788608862 (ebook)

EU GPSR representative: LOGOS EUROPE, 9 rue Nicolas Poussin, LA ROCHELLE 17000, France Contact@logoseurope.eu

Want to bulk-buy copies of this book for your team and colleagues? We can customize the content and co-brand *The Wellbeing Advantage* to suit your business's needs.

Please email info@practicalinspiration.com for more details.

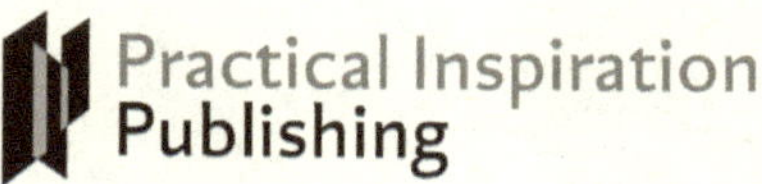

Contents

Foreword

In my years practising as a general practitioner and specializing in lifestyle medicine, I've witnessed first hand how small, consistent shifts in habits can transform a person's health. Our modern lives are full of conflicting demands: work pressures, family responsibilities, digital distractions, and the constant pull of convenience. It is in this complexity that true wellbeing doesn't happen by chance; it must be consciously designed.

This book arrives at a vital time in the wellbeing conversation. It doesn't promise quick fixes. Instead, it offers something far more valuable: a pathway to sustained progress and how we can build habits that endure, adapt to change, and build a foundation for a healthier future.

From my perspective, three pillars define the strength of Janine's approach: wearable technology, self-reflection through journalling, and habit architecture for lasting change.

Firstly, wearable technology gives us a window into our bodies that we've never had before. Smartwatches and fitness trackers, when used intelligently, can become instruments to support self-awareness. They can help us stay motivated, understand more about how our body works, identify recovery gaps, and give us measurable data to track progress. Wearing a tracker and reviewing the data becomes not a chore but a motivation for sustained progress.

Secondly, self-reflection forms the mirror to those insights. Data without context can mislead. Journalling adds meaning, helping us notice patterns, triggers, and emotional shifts that influence health. Janine's framework for reflection encourages curiosity over criticism: *Why did I sleep poorly last night?* or *What caused this rise in resting heart rate?* Over time, this dialogue between data and reflection becomes a personal feedback loop where you measure, understand, and recalibrate your next step.

Thirdly, habits don't change by force; they evolve through design. This book shows how to create routines that align with your values, energy, and environment. It moves beyond guilt-based resolutions to promote layered, incremental progress, stacking micro-habits, and allowing space for course corrections. People thrive when they stop viewing change as a battle of willpower and start seeing it as a system designed for real life.

What this book ultimately offers is a bridge between scientific evidence and lived experience. It reframes wellbeing as something dynamic, a negotiation between structure and flexibility, performance and recovery, striving and self-compassion.

To the reader: I highly suspect you already care about your health. But converting that into a lifestyle that promotes health in our modern environment is challenging, but possible! This book is a guide, grounded in science and empathy. Use it as you would a trusted adviser: experiment, reflect, and iterate. The path to lasting wellbeing isn't linear, but with these frameworks, you'll be equipped to navigate its turns with confidence.

May *The Wellbeing Advantage* guide you to weave data and reflection into your daily life, shaping habits that sustain your energy, deepen your awareness, and support your wellbeing for years to come.

Dr Hussain Al-Zubaidi
Lifestyle GP, TV Doctor,
RCGP Lifestyle & Physical Activity Champion

Reader's guide

This book is an invitation to explore, experiment, and build a personalized wellbeing toolkit; one that fits the realities of a busy professional life. Together, we'll lay the foundation for small, daily habits that sustain not just your work, but your whole life.

How this book helps. The habits here can meaningfully improve overall wellbeing, supporting energy, recovery, mood, and long-term health. The focus is preventative: small, consistent actions reduce future risk and enhance quality of life, whatever your starting point.

A brief note on scope. This is not a substitute for medical advice, diagnosis, or treatment. It does not replace personalized care for clinical conditions (for example, hormone imbalances, heart disease, diabetes, chronic illness, cancer, mental health disorders, or specialist dietary needs). If you are living with any of these or have severe or persistent symptoms, please seek advice from qualified health professionals.

Navigating hormone change. Variations across the monthly cycle, perimenopause, and menopause can influence energy, mood, and sleep. While this book isn't a clinical protocol, the habits inside help you navigate change with greater clarity, balance, and self-kindness.

Use the data; trust your body. Wearables offer helpful data points, not diagnoses. Treat the numbers as guides to notice patterns, build awareness, and make more informed choices around sleep, stress, movement, and recovery. Pair trends with brief pen-and-paper reflections on your energy, mood, focus, and capacity. Let data guide, and your body decide, with care, compassion, and confidence.

Introduction

Most days don't start with calm. The moment the alarm sounds, your mind floods with tasks to manage and things to remember. You're already on before you've even begun, reacting before you've had a chance to think. Your body feels it too: tight shoulders, shallow breath, and a rising sense of overwhelm that's hard to shake.

If that sounds familiar, you're far from alone. Burnout, exhaustion, and stress-related illness are on the rise; nearly one in three adults report high or extreme levels of pressure.[1] Most of us begin our days already under strain from a steady accumulation of small stresses that push our system into overdrive before we've even left the house. The way we're working and living is unsustainable. But it doesn't have to stay this way.

Here's the change: true wellbeing isn't about pushing through; it's about finding balance. When our days are planned with intention and paired with healthy habits, we give our body and mind what they need to thrive. We're not designed to run on empty; we're designed to recover, rebuild, and renew. When effort and recovery work together, energy stabilizes, focus sharpens, and wellbeing becomes our advantage.

This book translates that principle into seven simple habits: routine, movement, nutrition, balance, rest, connection, and sleep. Personalize them to your life, whether you're leading a team, running a business, or juggling work and home. Together we'll cut through the noise and focus on what truly supports your body and brain, helping you feel calmer, clearer, and able to sustain energy when it matters most.

No fads: just practical, evidence-based steps you can apply straight away. When you prioritize your wellbeing, you don't just get through the day; you create the conditions to thrive in work and life.

The spark behind *The Wellbeing Advantage*

When I began writing *The Wellbeing Advantage*, my goal was simple: to create the resource I wish I'd had during some of the most challenging periods of my own life. Like many of the professionals I now work with, I know what it's like to feel chronically fatigued, emotionally drained, and stretched to the point of breaking. I've lived through significant mental health challenges and the kind of debilitating fatigue that makes even small decisions too heavy to handle. This book is my answer to a question so many of us carry:

> *How can we build wellbeing into our day so it feels supportive, not like another thing on the to-do list?*

That question became the heart of my work, but the story started long before I became a wellbeing coach.

Where it all began

I've always been fascinated by what it takes to perform at your best. I grew up playing junior national tennis, immersed in a high-performance world of training, testing limits, and learning about movement, strength, nutrition, and mindset. That passion led me to a career in sport science, where I studied elite athletes, exploring how they sustain performance, build resilience, and recover under pressure.

My work took me to the All England Lawn Tennis Club Wimbledon, researching the life stories of female players competing both before and after the Second World War. Interviewing these inspiring women, including 1956 Wimbledon finalist Christine Truman, taught me something powerful: the lessons of high-performance sport don't just belong on the court. They can shape how we live, work, and recover across all stages of life.

Those lessons became deeply personal when my mental health deteriorated, and I experienced clinical depression first hand. No amount of knowledge could protect me from the reality of my own body and mind reaching their limits. But when I began to rebuild, everything I had learned from the world of elite sport, including recovery, nervous system regulation, and small, consistent habits became the foundation for my recovery.

That experience changed everything. Retraining as a transformational coach was the best decision I could have made, not just for myself and my family, but for the clients I now support. It gave me the clarity, purpose, and direction I'd been searching for. I wasn't starting over. I was finally building something that felt aligned. And now, I help others do the same, navigating change not by overhauling their lives, but by rebuilding from within.

From sport science to *The Wellbeing Advantage*

During my early career as a wellbeing coach, I often collaborated with my husband Ken, a high-performance sport scientist working with Olympic athletes. Together, we explored how wearable technology could monitor performance and recovery. I was fascinated by how this real-time data was being used, not just to track effort, but to guide smarter choices, manage recovery, and respond to stress with precision. It sparked a powerful question:

> *What if professionals outside of sport could access this kind of insight? What if my clients could see in real time how their choices were impacting their energy, focus, and capacity?*

That moment sharpened the focus of my work. I realized my role wasn't just to coach from the outside in, but to equip clients with the same kind of precision, insight, and sustainable performance strategies used in elite sport.

It was the perfect fusion of everything I'd spent my career learning, bringing together transformational coaching, mindset, behavioural science, and physiology. It meant supporting clients from the inside out, combining personalized data with science-backed habits that create meaningful, lasting change.

Since then, I've worked with hundreds of professionals, from senior leaders and midlife career changers, to founders, and people at a crossroads in their work, health, or life. Many arrive already doing all the *right* things: reading the books, listening to the podcasts, and trying the latest wellbeing trends. Yet they still feel stuck, inundated with advice, and unsure what will really work for *their* body, mind, and life.

You're not alone if you've wondered

- *Why am I still exhausted, even though I'm trying to do all the right things?*
- *What's draining me and what will help me recover, without overhauling my life?*
- *How can I tell what my body needs right now?*

Your seven transformative habits

Through my work, I've identified seven transformative habits that stand out as the real game changers: routine, movement, nutrition, balance, rest, connection, and sleep.

I call them habits because they aren't one-off strategies, they're small, repeatable actions you can weave into your life until they become part of who you are. They're transformative because they shift how you feel, think, and show up in the world, not through willpower, but through consistency and alignment.

These habits reflect the principles of transformational coaching, where deep, sustainable change happens not by doing more, but by building practices that are rooted in self-awareness and aligned with what matters most to you.

On their own, each habit strengthens a key aspect of your health, energy, and resilience. Together, they create a holistic, sustainable approach that lets you perform at your best without sacrificing your health, focus, or peace of mind.

Small steps, big wins

- **Your Routine Habit**: optimize your morning routine to boost energy, focus, and control, setting the tone for the rest of your day.
- **Your Movement Habit**: discover how to weave movement into busy schedules to lift vitality, mood, and long-term health.
- **Your Nutrition Habit**: fuel your body and brain with simple nutrition and hydration strategies that stabilize energy and sharpen thinking.
- **Your Balance Habit**: find your rhythm between focus and recovery, staying effective without losing yourself to stress.
- **Your Rest Habit**: reset and recharge with micro-breaks and science-based pauses that protect energy and restore clarity.
- **Your Connection Habit**: nurture meaningful connections that buffer stress, energize you, and strengthen resilience.
- **Your Sleep Habit**: reclaim restorative sleep to repair your body, restore your mind, and leave you waking refreshed.

From survival to sustainable success

Real transformation isn't about doing more; it's about regaining clarity, confidence, and control.

This shift takes you from running on empty to feeling grounded. From reactive, overstretched days to intentional ones. From wondering what's wrong to understanding what your body is really telling you and knowing how to respond.

Transformation means recognizing the early-warning signs of **burnout**, not just mentally or emotionally but physically. These signs can be subtle, revealed through wearables or reflection, sometimes even before you're consciously aware of them. As you tune in, you begin to understand what your stress responses look and feel like, and how to intervene before the pressure gets too much. This awareness allows you to protect your energy without guilt, create breathing space without losing momentum, and make decisions rooted in wellbeing, not obligation.

It's not about becoming a different person. It's about returning to a calm, focused, capable version of yourself; one that can live, lead, and perform sustainably without compromising your health.

It's not just about living longer, it's about living better

Living better for longer is often described as 'healthspan' a term introduced by physician and longevity expert Peter Attia.[2] It refers not just to how long you live, but to the number of years you remain healthy, active, and fully functional.

Extending your healthspan comes down to small, daily choices. These seemingly minor habits shape not only how long you live, but how well you live; physically, mentally, and emotionally.

Many people still think wellbeing is simply the absence of illness, or that it starts and ends with diet, exercise, and sleep. True wellbeing goes further. It includes how you manage your energy, how you recover, and how you think, feel, and connect with others. It's not about doing more; it's about making what you already do work better for you.

Scientific research backs this up: people with higher levels of wellbeing don't just feel better, they live longer, experience fewer health problems, and perform better under pressure.[3] Sounds like something we should all get on board with.

Reflection moment

How are your daily choices shaping not just the length of your life, but the quality of the years you're living?

The rise of wearables for wellbeing

Wearable technology, like smartwatches and fitness trackers, has gradually become part of everyday life. It can be a powerful ally when it comes to tracking your progress and tuning into what your body truly needs. Whether you wear a smartwatch or carry a smartphone that tracks your steps, chances are you're already collecting data about your body. From tracking sleep patterns to monitoring heart rate and daily movement, these devices provide meaningful insights, making the impact of everyday strain visible in real time and confirming what your body already knows: something has to change.

No wearable? No problem

If you don't use a wearable, stay with me. The strategies in this book stand on their own to help you build habits that last. Data can help you personalize and refine them, but it isn't essential. The real advantage comes from small, consistent actions you can start today, with or without a device.

The future of health is wearable

In the UK, the adoption of wearable health technology is rapidly rising, with about 30–40% of adults using wearable devices regularly.[4] Yet despite the growing popularity, many users still don't fully engage with the advanced health and performance-tracking features available.[5] Devices are worn, data is collected, but often, no action is taken. If this sounds familiar, it's not on you, it just means you need clearer guidance and a simpler plan.

And that's where this book comes in. The aim isn't to turn you into a data analyst, but to demystify wearable data and show you how to use it as a tool for insightful, sustainable change. Whether you're tracking sleep, movement, or stress, wearable devices can reveal patterns you might otherwise miss, patterns that help you build better habits and catch early signs of burnout before they spiral.

A rising heart rate, restless nights, and low recovery scores aren't just numbers; they're your body's early-warning system before burnout hits. On the flip side, sustained energy, restorative sleep, and manageable stress are your cues to keep doing what works.

Reflection moment

If your wearable could speak, would it be urging you to slow down, or celebrating how far you've come?

Demystifying the data

Your wearable doesn't just track generic data, it captures personalized insights that reflect your unique physiology, lifestyle, and daily demands. Think of it as a mirror, helping you see what's really going on beneath the surface.

That's why it's unhelpful to compare your heart rate, sleep scores, or step count with someone else. Their body, activity levels, and stress responses are different from yours. The real power of wearable technology lies in its ability to reflect *your* trends over time. By consistently measuring your progress against yourself, you can spot patterns, recognize early signs of strain, and make informed adjustments.

While no consumer device is perfect, it's worth noting that although wearables may be slightly less accurate than laboratory-grade tools, they are highly consistent in how they track your own trends over time. When you use the same device at the same time each day, you gain reliable feedback that reflects your body's response, not just on one day, but across weeks and months.

Before you go any further, let's pause and explore the core metrics themselves. Understanding what your device is really telling you is the first step to putting that data to work for you.

Resting and real-time heart rate

Your heart rate is one of the most accessible and insightful physiological signals your body gives you. Most wearables track two key metrics: **resting heart rate** (RHR) and **real-time heart rate**. Together, they offer a powerful window into your fitness, recovery, and day-to-day resilience. RHR is the average number of times your heart beats per minute when at rest. It's usually calculated by tracking pulse signals when you've been inactive or relaxed for several minutes. A lower RHR typically indicates better cardiovascular health, improved endurance, and a well-recovered body. Tracking RHR over time can help detect early signs of stress, illness, or poor sleep, empowering you to adjust your workload or recovery plans.

How to measure your RHR

1. **Choose the right time**: the best time to check your RHR is first thing in the morning, before getting out of bed, while still lying down. This is when your body is most at rest.

2. **Find your pulse**: place your index and middle fingers on your radial artery (inside of the wrist) or carotid artery (left side of the neck).
3. **Count beats**: count the number of beats for 60 seconds using a stopwatch or timer. I usually count for 30 seconds and multiply by 2.
4. **Repeat over three–five mornings**: for accuracy, take an average across several days.

For context, elite endurance athletes' RHR may be as low as 35–45 beats per minute (bpm). A healthy RHR ranges between 50 and 80 bpm for adults, but what matters most is your personal baseline over time, not a single reading. Always combine wearable data with body awareness: how you feel matters as much as what your tracker reports.

Real-time heart rate, on the other hand, shows how your heart responds moment to moment, whether you're exercising, in a meeting, stuck in traffic, or winding down in the evening. Many wearables now use real-time heart rate to estimate strain, energy levels, and training zones, giving you a real-time reflection of how external pressures are affecting your internal state.

Used together, your RHR and real-time heart rate help you go beyond numbers to meaningful insight. They're not just metrics, they're messages. When you start listening, you can respond with intention, not just reaction.

Step count and activity monitoring

Step count data helps assess daily activity levels, sedentary time, and calorie expenditure. Most wearables use a combination of motion sensors, including gyroscopes and accelerometers, to track daily steps, estimate energy expenditure, and prompt you to break up long periods of sitting.

But steps alone don't tell the full story. Many wearables also track activity intensity and overall load giving insight not just into how much you moved, but how hard your body was working. Load reflects both volume (how long you moved) and intensity (how hard you worked), helping you understand the impact movement has on your energy, recovery, and progress over time.

Sleep duration and quality

Most wearables provide insights into how long you sleep and how restorative that sleep is. These insights are typically summarized in a sleep score or sleep performance rating, which combines factors including total time asleep, time in bed, how long it took you to fall asleep, and your amount of **deep sleep** and **REM sleep** (rapid eye movement: the stage where most dreaming occurs). Some devices also track sleep regularity, restlessness, and your body's overall recovery. These scores give you a picture of how well-rested you truly are, not just how long you were in bed.

Sleep insights from your wearable

- **Sleep score**: a single score summarizing your total sleep duration and quality.
- **Sleep stages**: time spent in light, deep, and REM sleep.
- **Sleep efficiency**: percentage of time spent asleep.
- **Sleep latency**: how long it took you to fall asleep.

That said, it's worth understanding the limits of your device. Wearables track sleep by monitoring movement and heart rate, whereas the gold standard, polysomnography, directly measures brainwaves, along with breathing, eye movements, and muscle activity. Your device won't label every stage with clinical precision, but it can still give a useful snapshot of your overall sleep and recovery patterns.

Think of your wearable as a personal guide not a diagnostic tool. Its real value lies in helping you spot trends, reflect on your sleep habits, and notice when your body needs more recovery.

Heart rate variability

People often imagine their heart rate as a metronome, beating at a constant steady rhythm. You may be surprised to hear that the time between heartbeats varies from one beat to the next, even when your heart rate appears consistent. This variation is called **heart rate variability (HRV)**. It's a core input that feeds into your wearable dashboard. A healthy heart is not perfectly regular, and this variability reflects how dynamically your body is adapting to both physical and emotional demands.

HRV is shaped by your **autonomic nervous system**, the part of your nervous system that runs automatically in the background, controlling things like breathing, digestion, and your stress response. This system balances two key branches: **sympathetic activation**, often described as the 'fight-or-flight' response, and **parasympathetic recovery**, your 'rest and digest' mode. In general, lower HRV aligns with higher stress load, while higher HRV reflects stronger recovery capacity.

It's not a simple on/off switch, but HRV provides a powerful lens into how effectively your body is shifting between these states. When your nervous system can fluidly shift states, you feel energized, resilient, and clear-headed.

Subtle drops in HRV can act as a helpful early warning, prompting you to adjust your movement, protect sleep, or prioritize recovery before you feel depleted. When your system gets stuck in high alert or in a flattened, shutdown mode, it's harder to think clearly, recover effectively, or feel fully yourself. Emerging frameworks also describe additional defence responses such as 'freeze or fawn', that can show up when the nervous system is under chronic pressure.[6]

Most wearables estimate HRV using photoplethysmography (PPG) sensors which use light to detect blood volume changes at the skin's surface. This allows you to monitor daily fluctuations and adjust your habits in response to signs of strain, not just after you feel depleted, but before.

There's no one-size-fits-all *ideal* HRV number. A healthy HRV can range anywhere from 20 to 120 milliseconds, depending on your age, fitness level, genetics, measurement method, and even the time of day. What matters most is your personal baseline, built from consistent readings (often after sleep) and over time. Many devices form an initial baseline after ~2–4 weeks of regular wear and keep refining it as more data accumulates. Expect your baseline to shift with extended stress, heavy training, illness, or disrupted sleep.

HRV is your body's inner dashboard explaining *why* you feel a certain way. Your baseline is the anchor; your trend is the signal. Don't chase daily swings, watch how your HRV shifts over 7–14 days relative to your baseline then course-correct your effort and recovery accordingly.

Daily readiness score

Your **readiness score** is your nervous system's performance review, telling you *how* much your body and nervous system have to give today. It doesn't care what's on your calendar, it reflects what your system can realistically handle.

Think of your readiness score as a summary metric. Instead of relying on one signal in isolation, your device blends multiple inputs, including heart rate, RHR, movement, sleep, and HRV, to give you a snapshot of your current state. In simple terms, it's the battery widget on your dashboard.

As Andrew Huberman, professor of neuroscience at Stanford University and host of the *Huberman Lab* podcast explains, these metrics act as 'real-time feedback loops'.[7] They don't just measure your habits, they reveal how your internal systems, especially your nervous system and recovery processes, are adapting under pressure.

Depending on your device, you might see this expressed as a readiness, recovery, or stress management score. A higher score suggests you're well recovered and primed for focus, activity, or challenge. A lower score is your body's way of asking for rest, lighter movement, or a more compassionate pace for the day ahead.

What makes your readiness score so powerful is that it doesn't just reflect physical exertion, it also accounts for emotional stress, poor sleep, travel, alcohol, and overstimulation. That makes it a powerful early-warning indicator, helping you spot depletion early and respond with intention, not just habit.

Caution: Data overload!

For many of my clients, wearable technology acts like a mirror, reflecting the truth of how their body is coping beneath the surface. The digital insights provide them with an X-ray of their day: a real-time view of how work, environment, sleep, stress, and routines affect capacity. And that insight is powerful. It shows how your body is really responding to pressure, where recovery is missing, and what your nervous system is telling you that your mind may be too busy to notice.

The number one drawback of wearable devices isn't the technology itself; it's how easily you can become obsessed with the data. While wearables are designed to support better decisions and a healthier life, having them on your body 24/7 makes it tempting to over-analyse every number. It's important to remember: your wearable reflects what you do, feel, and experience.

The data mirrors your reality; it doesn't define it. One night of poor sleep or a dip in readiness doesn't mean you've failed; it's your body offering feedback. What matters most is the pattern over time. This book will help you interpret your data with a longer-term lens, integrating what the data shows with how you *feel*, so you can make smart, compassionate choices that support your wellbeing.

You might wake up feeling refreshed, until you check your wearable, see a poor sleep score, and suddenly start questioning how you feel. This is where there's a risk you become what's known as the 'worried well'.

The 'worried well' refers to people who are generally healthy yet seek intervention and medical advice due to concerns about potential illness. They often experience heightened anxiety about their health even in the absence of significant medical symptoms. Constant tracking of metrics like heart rate, sleep, or readiness scores can lead to obsessive behaviours or unnecessary worry. Striking a balance between using your wearable for empowerment versus over-reliance is key to avoiding these pitfalls.

How to use this book

The book is designed to follow the natural rhythm of your day, starting with how you wake up and ending with how you wind down. Ideally, you'll read it in order, flowing with the rhythm of your day. But if one area feels especially relevant right now, whether it's sleep, rest, connection, or movement, feel free to start there. This isn't a rigid programme; it's a flexible framework to meet you where you are.

Reflection moments

Each chapter includes regular prompts to help you pause, reset, and apply what you've learned. These reflection moments are designed to help you recognize patterns in your energy, stress responses, and daily capacity.

Keep a pen and notebook nearby, use your journal, an app, or even voice notes, whatever helps you engage with the ideas and tune into your own wellbeing. This isn't just about reading, it's about listening in and making small, intentional adjustments that steadily change how you feel, think, and perform.

Real client stories

You'll meet clients, people just like you, who've moved from burnout to balance by creating simple, science-based habits aligned with their values and their lives. All stories are drawn from my client work, though names and identifying details have been changed to protect confidentiality.

Your wearable, your data

If you wear a smartwatch or use trackers and wearable health devices, you'll find specific guidance in each chapter on how to harness data from your wearable device. You'll be able to personalize your habits, spot early signs of strain, and make smarter decisions that support your energy, focus, and long-term wellbeing.

But if wearables aren't for you, that's absolutely fine. You can still gain powerful insights by tuning into your body's natural rhythms using the tools woven throughout the book, especially the 'Aha Model' which is designed for everyone.

The Aha Model: A framework for change

Each chapter culminates in my evidence-backed 'Aha Model', a simple, science-informed process to turn self-awareness into habit change. The model mirrors the moment in transformational coaching when a client experiences that powerful shift: an 'aha' moment of clarity about what truly matters and what to do next.

Whether you're guided by technology, personal insight, or both, the 'Aha Model' invites you to pause, reflect, and apply the core principles of behaviour change to turn awareness into aligned action.

The Aha Model

1. **Awareness**: this is where change begins. Pause to notice what's happening in your life right now. What feels out of sync? What would you like to improve? Awareness shifts you from autopilot to intentional action.
2. **Habit**: identify one small, practical step that aligns with your values, lifestyle, and overall wellbeing goals. Using reflective coaching questions, you'll choose a habit that feels meaningful, realistic, and sustainable.
3. **Action**: finally, you bring it to life. Through approaches like habit stacking, behaviour cues, and micro-shifts, you'll embed the new habit into your daily routine, in a way that sticks, without adding pressure.

Your roadmap to *The Wellbeing Advantage*

When it comes to wellbeing, it's tempting to focus on just one piece of the puzzle, maybe improving your sleep, managing stress, or increasing movement, while unintentionally neglecting the rest. But true wellbeing is holistic. When one part of your health is out of sync, it affects everything else: your energy, focus, mood, performance, and the quality of your relationships.

That's why this book doesn't offer a one-size-fits-all plan. Instead, it gives you a flexible framework to experiment, reflect, and refine, until healthy habits become second nature. This isn't about chasing perfection. It's about creating progress you can feel through small, intentional changes that align with your life, energy, and values. Let's begin where every healthy day starts, with an effective, consistent routine that works for you.

1

Your Routine Habit

Most of us don't leap out of bed feeling refreshed, clear-headed, and fully in control. More often, the day starts with a familiar hum of chaos: managing family logistics, choosing what to wear, rushing to prepare for a client presentation, or scrolling through overnight emails before even making it to the kettle. These small, cumulative pressures, known as micro-stresses, chip away at your focus and energy before the day has even begun. While they might seem insignificant in isolation, these early stressors can set the tone for everything that follows, nudging you into a reactive state where you're chasing the day instead of leading it.

But it doesn't have to be that way. A simple repeatable morning routine can change the whole trajectory of your day by reducing micro-stresses and setting you up for a day that flows smoothly, with less stress and more ease. When your mornings begin with intention rather than urgency, you calm the nervous system, minimize unnecessary choices, and regain a sense of control even when the rest of the day is unpredictable.

The invisible cost of a chaotic morning

Ever felt groggy mid-morning, even after a full night's sleep? Or noticed your energy crashing earlier than expected? It might not be about how many hours you slept, but about how your day began.

A chaotic morning isn't just a passing inconvenience; it sets the tone for the entire day. Studies show that professionals with structured routines experience lower anxiety and greater workplace satisfaction.[1] By contrast, professionals who consistently start their day without structure experience higher levels of stress-related inflammation,[2] lower work engagement and satisfaction, and an increased risk of burnout.[3]

Many professionals unknowingly set themselves up for stress by beginning their day chasing tasks instead of setting priorities. In a busy household, preparing for work, managing early tasks, perhaps getting children ready for school, can feel like a race against the clock. Think about how many small decisions you make before you even start your workday: what to wear, what to eat, when to leave, and how to respond to unread emails. These small, repeated pressures accumulate as micro-stress doses, gradually eroding your sense of calm.[4]

You don't need a complete change in lifestyle to shift your morning habits. Small, strategic changes can have an immediate and lasting impact. Strategies such as delaying digital distractions, incorporating movement, ensuring proper nutrition, and prioritizing exposure to natural light help recalibrate your brain, setting the tone for a more productive and focused day.

In this chapter, you'll see how a simple morning routine can create meaningful shifts in wellbeing and performance. You'll unpack the science of habit formation, examine how positive psychology supports routines that last, and find help to build a personalized start to the day that fits your needs. You'll also meet Remi, whose story illustrates how small, consistent changes restore calm, clarity, and a sense of control.

By the end, you'll understand why routines matter and how to craft sustainable morning habits, regardless of whether you have wearable technology or not. You'll gain insights that help you tune into the natural rhythms of your body to optimize your daily start. Whether you're balancing career and family, working remotely, or refocusing on your wellbeing, you'll leave with practical tools to build resilience and support you through the challenges of daily life.

Meet Remi: Under pressure before 9 a.m.

Remi is 45 years old and a senior operations manager in a fast-growing tech company. She is known for her sharp thinking, calmness under pressure, and ability to get things done. On the surface, her life looks ideal: a career on the rise, a strong reputation among colleagues, and a busy home life shared with her partner and two teenage boys. Yet beneath it all, the steady build-up of everyday stresses is starting to catch up with her. She no longer feels fully in control; it's starting to feel like too much.

Each morning Remi wakes already anxious, dreading the flood of unread emails. She barely has time to process her thoughts before diving into work demands. Skipping breakfast is the norm, and as she frantically throws on an outfit, her mind races ahead to a day of back-to-back meetings. The stress is unrelenting, making her feel like she is always playing catch-up. By the time she reaches her desk, her chest feels tight, her thinking foggy, and her patience thin.

Though she continues to show up and meet expectations, the strain is beginning to show. The constant pressure is starting to erode both her confidence and the quality of her work. Simple tasks feel overwhelming. She is second-guessing emails, hesitating in meetings, and responding curtly to colleagues. She is aware of her irritability but can't seem to shake it. By midday, Remi relies on caffeine to mask the fatigue that simmers beneath the surface. At night, she goes to bed exhausted, replaying the unfinished tasks in her mind, dreading the same cycle repeating the next day. The feeling of being constantly *on* is draining her, but she has no idea how to break the cycle.

Through the course of our work together Remi makes simple but powerful shifts to her mornings. She stops reaching for her phone the moment she wakes up. Instead, she begins each day with a small ritual: stepping outside for 15 minutes of morning light. At first it feels forced, but soon the fresh air and natural light become the anchor of her day.

Instead of diving straight into her inbox, she pauses to write down her top three priorities for the day. That pause gives her a sense of control before the demands of others take over. Once her new morning routine is established, she introduces additional habits: a glass of water to hydrate, a few minutes of light stretching to awaken her body, and together these shifts create a calmer, more intentional start to the day.

The impact is remarkable. Within weeks, Remi's energy stabilizes, her stress levels drop, and her mornings shift from frantic to focused. Meetings become more productive. Her decision-making sharpens. Her interactions soften. She isn't just getting through the morning; she's leading it.

Remi's story shows just how powerful a structured routine can be, not just for performance, but for reclaiming a sense of calm and control. And she's not alone. Many of my clients start their day in a state of reaction, scanning headlines, checking messages, and rushing through routines. But this comes at a cost: rising stress, decision fatigue, and a steady erosion of focus and emotional resilience.

By examining the invisible toll of chaotic mornings, you see how small changes in how you start the day can build a powerful foundation that leaves you feeling in control and ready for the day ahead.

Reflection moment

Does your morning begin by design or by default?

What's one small change you could make tomorrow morning to feel more grounded, clear, or in control before the day takes over?

Reset your mornings for success

Your body runs on an internal clock known as the **circadian rhythm**, a 24-hour cycle that regulates everything from your energy and mood to your hormone levels and focus. And this clock relies heavily on one key signal: light. Without this natural signal, your internal clock struggles to stay on track and you feel sluggish, foggy, and prone to energy dips as the day goes on.

Morning light sets the rhythm

When morning light reaches your eyes, it sends a powerful signal to your brain that sets the tone for the day ahead. Light cues your body to suppress **melatonin**, the hormone that supports sleep, while increasing **cortisol** to boost alertness and **serotonin** to lift mood and stabilize energy. This natural sequence helps your body shift from night to day, priming you to feel awake, focused, and ready to go.[5]

When people think of cortisol, they often associate it with stress and with good reason. But cortisol isn't always the villain and shouldn't be avoided altogether. In fact, it plays a vital role in keeping you alert, focused, and energized, especially first thing in the morning. This natural rise in cortisol helps regulate your circadian rhythm, sets your energy for the next 16 hours, and prepares you physiologically for alertness and decision-making.

In contrast, when cortisol peaks too late in the day due to insufficient morning light, overstimulation, or poor sleep, it can delay melatonin production, disrupt sleep quality, and throw your entire biological rhythm off track. Remember, the goal isn't to eliminate cortisol, but to get the timing right: you want cortisol to rise early, peak in the morning, and taper off as evening approaches.

Morning light is especially important for professionals working in office environments with little access to natural light.[6] Over time, waking in the dark, scrolling indoors, and diving straight into tasks without seeing daylight chips away at energy, clarity, and emotional regulation. If stepping outdoors isn't immediately possible, even sitting near a window or stepping onto a balcony can help your brain receive this vital environmental cue.

In a world where you spend so much time indoors, reconnecting with morning light may be one of the simplest, and most accessible ways to boost your wellbeing, starting right from the moment your day begins.

Reflection moment

Tomorrow morning, could your first steps be outside in natural light? Notice how it changes your mood, focus, and energy for the rest of the day.

Switch on with morning movement

Exposure to natural light, combined with light movement such as a short jog, walk, or gentle stretch, helps synchronize your body clock, boost mood through **dopamine** and serotonin, and sharpen focus for the day. Stepping outside for 15 minutes in the morning was revolutionary for Remi. It's not about getting up three hours earlier or hitting the gym at dawn; it's about developing a morning routine that calms the chaos and sharpens your senses for the day ahead.

Reclaim your morning from screens

If your first act in the morning is to reach for your phone for email or news updates, you're forcing your brain to deal with multiple cognitive tasks before it's fully prepared. This early-morning multitasking overloads working memory, triggers the brain's stress response system, and makes it harder to engage in deep, meaningful work.[7] Instead of easing into the day with clarity, you start in a state of information overload. That early flood of data lingers, making it harder to concentrate and process tasks effectively.

Put simply, your ability to make high-quality decisions declines as the day goes on.[8] Every choice, big or small, draws on the same finite mental resource. That's why streamlining your mornings is so powerful. By removing decisions, like choosing what to wear or what to have for breakfast, you preserve cognitive energy for the choices that matter most.

Recognizing the value of having a morning routine is the first step in making meaningful changes to regain control and cultivate a sense of balance and preparedness from the moment your day begins. By streamlining your morning routine and replacing digital distractions with mindful habits, your cognitive resources are preserved for high-value work rather than dissipated on trivial choices, leading to greater cognitive resilience over time. When you recognize the cost of chaotic mornings and take steps to reset your routine, you don't just transform the way you start your day, you change how you experience your entire life.

Now that you've looked at the benefits of a morning routine, it's time to explore how to make new habits stick. Because noticing what helps is only part of the story, the real transformation happens when those helpful routines become automatic.

Routines that stick

There's a wealth of brilliant research out there on the science of behaviour change, each theory offering a slightly different lens on what makes habits last. If you're curious to dig deeper, I've included a selection of additional texts in the 'Further reading' section. For building routines that work in real life, especially under pressure, I've chosen techniques that have consistently delivered results for my clients. They've been tested, reviewed, and refined in fast-paced environments, and I'm confident they can work for you too.

The power of tiny habits

Even with the best intentions, habits don't always take hold. If you've ever started a new routine only to abandon it weeks later, you're not the only one. The frustration of failed habits often leads people to believe they lack discipline, but research shows that habit formation is not about discipline or willpower, it's about strategy. After decades studying human behaviour at Stanford University, B.J. Fogg discovered something simple yet profound: the secret to lasting change isn't willpower; it's starting small.[9]

Small, consistent actions may seem insignificant day-to-day, but when repeated, they create powerful shifts in identity, capability, and long-term wellbeing. It's not about dramatic overnight change, it's about building momentum through achievable, repeatable wins.

The science of tiny habits

In his book *Tiny Habits*, Fogg shows that meaningful change starts small. New behaviours stick when you anchor them to something you already do, perform them in a tiny, almost effortless way, and celebrate immediately. This three-part structure, **anchor**, **behaviour**, **celebration**, is the foundation of building an effective routine that works with your brain's natural habit machinery. Once a habit forms, the brain runs on autopilot. It stops participating in decision-making and performs automatically, conserving energy by removing the need for conscious decision-making.

How tiny habits take hold

1. **Anchor**: tie the new habit to a behaviour you already do consistently (like brushing your teeth or boiling the kettle).
2. **Behaviour**: introduce the new habit but keep it tiny, almost laughably small. For example, add just two squats to your morning routine.
3. **Celebration**: reinforce it emotionally with a positive reaction. You can smile, fist pump, or say '*Yes!*' to trigger a dopamine release.

Fogg's model complements Charles Duhigg's habit loop, outlined in his book *The Power of Habit* which breaks habit formation into **cue**, **routine**, **reward**.[10] The cue is a trigger that initiates the habit, the routine is the behaviour you perform in response, and the reward is the benefit your brain learns to expect. Together, these frameworks show how habits form, and how to disrupt unhelpful routines and design better ones, starting with something as small as stepping outside each morning.

The key idea running through both models is that your brain doesn't distinguish between habits that help or harm, it repeats whatever you give it. That's why the small choices you prioritize each morning matter so much. Build routines that energize, ground, and move you closer to the life you want, because once they're in place, your brain will keep them on repeat.

Rewiring routine: How Remi created change

To illustrate this in real life, let's return to Remi. Her original morning routine looked like this: the anchor was waking up and feeling under pressure. The behaviour that followed was reaching for her phone to scroll through emails, seeking reassurance or a sense of control. Her celebration was a temporary dopamine hit from feeling on top of things, but this left her more anxious and reactive in the long term, rather than grounded.

Remi recognized that this habit was negatively impacting her mood and productivity. Once she understood how habits were formed, she could identify the cue, waking up under pressure, and intentionally replace her response with a more effective habit. Instead of reaching for her phone, she placed a journal by her bedside and wrote down three priorities for the day. This new habit still satisfied the craving for clarity and reassurance but in a way that empowered her rather than drained her. Her reward was a sense of control and preparedness, reinforcing a productive and positive start to her day.

This is the power of understanding habit formation: once you identify your cues, you can actively reshape your response and reinforce a new habit that serves you, rather than one that diminishes your wellbeing. You can replace small, unhelpful habits in your morning routine with intentional choices that set you up for a more focused, energized day.

Reflection moment

What's one habit you'd like to let go of and what could you replace it with?

Train your brain for positivity

A crucial element of behaviour change is **mindset**. If you believe that improving your wellbeing is difficult, time-consuming, or unsustainable, you'll struggle to make changes stick. But by shifting your mindset, focusing on small, achievable wins, you begin to rewire your brain to embrace positive change.

One striking example is 'the Tetris effect'. Tetris is a classic puzzle video game, where players rotate and arrange falling geometric shapes, called 'tetrominoes', to complete and clear horizontal lines before the screen fills up. After extended play, people began seeing the game's patterns in real life, automatically looking for ways to fit shapes together.[11]

Harvard-trained positive psychology researcher and bestselling author Shawn Achor has expanded on this idea. He found that when you consistently focus on positive habits and moments, your brain becomes primed to seek out and reinforce those patterns.[12] Just as Tetris players start seeing the game's shapes everywhere, people who adopt a positive mindset start noticing more opportunities to support their habits. It's not just a cognitive shift; it's a way of training your brain to work for you, not against you.

Prime positivity with gratitude

Gratitude creates a positive Tetris effect. By logging small positives (a kind message, a great coffee, a quiet commute) you train attention towards what's positive. Over time your brain gets better at finding those pieces that 'fit', which boosts motivation and optimism and makes healthy choices easier.[13] By practising gratitude regularly, you prime your brain to keep finding the pieces that fit, making it more likely you'll see (and take) chances to move, rest, and connect.

Try this:

1. **Three good things**: each morning, note three specific positives from the last 24 hours.
2. **Focus on the why**: add a short 'because... ' to deepen the memory and make it stick.
3. **Spot an opportunity**: finish with one tiny action that builds on those positives (e.g. send a quick thank you to someone who helped yesterday).

Rigidity kills routine success

If you expect your morning routine to be flawless from day one, you set yourself up for disappointment. Instead, embrace a flexible, progress-over-perfection mindset. Wendy Wood, one of the world's leading experts on the psychology of habits and professor of behavioural science, reminds us that true habit formation allows room for occasional breaks without derailing progress.[14]

Perfectionist thinking sets unrealistic expectations, causing routines to fail if they prove unsustainable. Yet life rarely follows a predictable path; unexpected challenges, responsibilities, and opportunities constantly arise. That's why it's so important to approach your routine with flexibility and self-compassion. Being adaptable allows you to stay aligned with your goals without feeling discouraged when things don't go as planned.

For example, if your morning routine includes a 20-minute workout but your schedule becomes more demanding, adjusting it to a 5-minute light stretching routine or yoga instead of dropping it entirely, helps sustain the habit. Adaptability increases habit longevity, making it easier to maintain routines despite changing circumstances.

Turn insights into action

Many people don't know where to start when adopting a new routine, whether you're working remotely, balancing a career and family, or struggling with getting up in the morning, the key is adapting habits to work for you.

Remote workers: Creating structure in a flexible environment

Working from home removes the natural transition between personal and professional life, which makes a structured morning even more essential. Without a commute, boundaries blur, focus slips, and motivation can dip.[15] Remote workers often find themselves lingering in a reactive state, checking emails first thing, and diving into tasks without mentally preparing for the day. That's why creating a morning routine that clearly signals the start of work is so vital when working remotely.

Small routines to structure your work-from-home day

- ✓ **Dress for work**: even if you work from home, changing into work clothes signals to your brain that the workday has begun.

- ✓ **Create a physical transition**: take a short walk or stretch before sitting at your desk to shift into a work mindset.
- ✓ **Time-block priorities**: start with structured deep work before checking emails to avoid falling into reaction mode.

Parents balancing career and family: Engage in small but powerful rituals

For parents, mornings are often dictated by the demands of family life, leaving little time for structured routines. Psychologist Barbara Fredrickson's research shows that parents who engage in micro-moments of mindfulness and movement experience lower stress levels and improved emotional resilience throughout the day.[16] It's easy to feel as if there's no space for self-care, but the key is to build small, sustainable habits rather than aiming for a rigid morning structure.

Morning routine tips for busy parents

- ✓ **Wake up before the household**: it may not feel great initially but even 10–15 minutes of quiet time before the morning rush can help set the tone for the day.
- ✓ **Incorporate children into small rituals**: a dance-off in the kitchen, preparing breakfast together, or setting daily intentions as a family can create shared habits that support both wellbeing and connection.
- ✓ **Leverage micro-moments**: when your morning is unpredictable, focus on one small habit that's non-negotiable, whether that's a few deep breaths, a hydration habit, or a quick stretch while your coffee brews.

Shift workers: Optimizing routine across changing schedules

One group often overlooked in discussions about morning routines are those whose schedules don't align with traditional work hours. Irregular sleep patterns and rotating work shifts disrupt the body's circadian rhythm, making structured routines more challenging. If you're working irregular hours, here are some habits to add to your routine to support your wellbeing.

Smart strategies for shift workers

- ✓ **Use bright light and movement**: signal the start of the day and help your body shift into wake mode.
- ✓ **Prioritize hydration, nutrition, and mindfulness**: build these into a simple wake-up ritual to stabilize energy and mood.
- ✓ **Stick to consistent sleep–wake patterns**: even on rest days, this helps regulate your body's internal clock.

Small, intentional changes don't just improve your morning, they transform how you experience your entire day, and wearable technology can help you notice the impact of these shifts in real time.

What your wearable tells you about Your Routine Habit

By tracking and interpreting wearable data, you can make informed decisions that help you start your day feeling energized and in control. The key is not just to collect data, but to actively use it to make simple, meaningful changes to your routine. When using a wearable device, consider the following key features when looking to improve your morning routine:

Resting heart rate

Monitoring resting heart rate (RHR) over time is a simple but powerful way to spot early signs that your body might be under strain. Low RHR in a well-recovered, energetic person is often a good sign of cardiovascular fitness, but if you feel drained, it's a signal to ease back and allow more recovery.

What to look for:

- Is your RHR elevated? You should adjust your morning routine to include hydration, deep breathing, and slower movement.
- Are you planning on adding exercise to your morning routine? It's worth checking your RHR to ensure your capacity for effort is there and you're not putting unnecessary strain on your body's resources.

Reflection moment

When you wake up is your RHR higher than usual?

Could your body be signalling the need for more recovery?

Sleep duration and quality insights

If you often wake feeling groggy, unfocused, or low on energy it's likely a consequence of poor sleep. You'll explore this more deeply in 'Your Sleep Habit', but for now, begin to track how changes to your morning routine influence how rested and ready you feel.

Rather than fixating on a single night's score, look for trends in your sleep over time by checking key sleep metrics such as sleep duration, and overall recovery scores.

A strong morning routine begins with one essential anchor: a consistent wake time. This simple habit plays a powerful role in regulating your circadian rhythm, which in turn supports stable sleep cycles. As your body clock becomes more aligned, you may start to notice improvements in total sleep duration and sleep quality scores which are essential for physical restoration, mental clarity, and emotional resilience.

What to look for:

- Sleep consistency: Are your bed and wake times roughly the same each day?
- Sleep efficiency: Do you fall asleep quickly and stay asleep?
- Sleep stages: Are you getting enough deep and REM (rapid eye movement) sleep to support full recovery?

Daily readiness score

If your wearable offers a daily readiness score, you can use it to adapt your morning routine more intentionally. It gives you a snapshot of how prepared your system is to perform; physically, mentally, and emotionally. Instead of guessing whether to push or pace yourself, readiness scores give you a science-backed guide for how to align your morning habits with your biology. It allows you to focus on what your body *needs* rather than what you *should* do.

What to look for:

- Is your daily readiness score lower than usual? This suggests you're not at full capacity. Begin the day with gentle movement, journalling, or meditation to ease into your day and delay intense work tasks until your energy improves later in the day.
- Is your morning readiness score higher than usual? This signals greater capacity for a productive, high-energy day.

Reflection moment

Based on your readiness score, what kind of morning routine would best serve you today: pushing forward, pacing yourself, or prioritizing recovery?

Now that you've explored the insights wearable technology can offer, let's shift towards an equally powerful, non-digital tool: self-reflection. While technology helps you *see* patterns, reflection helps you *understand* them.

Your routine breakthrough

Whether you use a wearable or not, journalling offers a powerful complement or alternative to data-driven routines. It helps you notice patterns, clarify intentions, and stay grounded. In a digital age, the act of writing things down brings a different kind of insight: personal, reflective, and deeply effective. By writing things down, you give your thoughts structure, your goals visibility, and your habits a place to take root.

Let's explore how to turn insights into action using the 'Aha Model' to unlock the morning routine that's right for you.

Awareness: Reflect on your current routine

Awareness is the first step. You can't change what you don't notice but once you do, small shifts become powerful. Imagine how different your day could feel if your morning set you up for success not stress.

Small shifts in your first hour can ripple across the day that follows. Use this morning energy check:

- Reflect on your energy levels upon waking: *Do you wake up feeling rested and ready, or sluggish and exhausted?*
- Notice your mindset and mental clarity: *Do you begin your day feeling clear-headed or already stressed and reactive?*
- Recognize your sense of control: *Do you feel in charge of your morning, or do external pressures dictate your start to the day?*

Habit: Identify the change that's needed

Simple habits with the power to transform your mornings include getting morning daylight, introducing light yoga stretches, or journalling. Identify your new morning habit by taking a few minutes to reflect and write your answers to the following prompts:

- *What's the very first thing you could do tomorrow morning that would make you feel more energized, grounded, or ready for the day ahead (e.g. sunlight, hydration, light movement)?*
- *Which new morning habit feels both realistic and meaningful to you right now?*
- *What could get in the way of this habit and what small adjustments could help it fit more smoothly in your day?*

Action: Sustaining your new routine

When it comes to building a habit, there's no magic number of days for the habit to stick. Despite the popular myth of 21 days, research shows there's no single number that works for everyone.[17] How long it takes for a new behaviour to feel automatic varies widely depending on the person, the behaviour, and the context. Some habits may feel natural within a few weeks, while others can take several months before they begin to feel automatic. What matters more than the exact number is how you design the habit itself. **Consistency**, **context**, and **simplicity** are the real drivers of success, the more repeatable and anchored your habit is, the more likely it is to last.[18]

As you already know from Fogg's 'Anchor-Behaviour-Celebration', the key to building an effective routine is not just to repeat it, but to *reward* it. Every time you celebrate your success, you trigger a release of dopamine. This dopamine response reinforces the neural pathways associated with the habit, increasing the likelihood you'll repeat the behaviour. Your brain is learning that this action matters and wants to do it again.

Reflection moment

Each morning, ask yourself: *How will I celebrate today's small win?*

Fredrickson's 'Broaden-and-Build Theory' supports this. Positive emotions don't just feel good; they widen your perspective and increase motivation, making you more likely to repeat productive behaviours and invest in long-term wellbeing.[19] When this happens, your brain tags the habit as valuable, setting you up to return to it, day after day.

Celebrate and reinforce your habit

- ✓ **Anchor it**: take a deep breath of fresh air and stretch your arms wide as you step outside; an instant anchor for your new habit.
- ✓ **Share it**: mention your new habit to your partner or a friend. Social accountability boosts emotional reward.
- ✓ **Savour it**: take a mindful moment to enjoy the feel of daylight and if you're lucky, maybe even the warmth of sun on your skin.

Master your mornings, master your life

Congratulations! You have added your first transformative habit to your wellbeing toolkit. You're on the path to transformation which you'll continue each morning as you intentionally set your day up for success.

The key to an effective morning routine isn't complexity, it's consistency. A sustainable routine is one that fits into your life, rather than forcing your life around it. By applying positive psychology principles, habit formation models, and incremental improvements, you can create a morning routine that promotes calm, boosts energy, and enhances long-term wellbeing.

By focusing on meaningful, personalized habits and leveraging behavioural science strategies, you can ensure that your morning routine becomes a natural, energizing part of your daily life, one that supports both professional success and personal wellbeing. Remi's journey demonstrates that transforming a chaotic morning doesn't require a massive overhaul, just intentional, strategic shifts. Whether you're a CEO, a remote worker, a parent, or a shift worker, the key is to design a routine that works for you.

Optimize your mornings

- ✓ **Step into natural light**: reset your circadian rhythm and lift your mood.
- ✓ **Add light movement**: wake up your body and sharpen mental alertness.
- ✓ **Hold off on technology**: give your brain space to wake naturally before diving into emails, messages, or news.
- ✓ **Practise gratitude**: direct your attention to what's positive and your brain will learn to find more of it, making positive choices feel easier and more natural.

2

Your Movement Habit

We were never designed to sit still all day, yet that's what modern work demands. Hours at a desk, endless video calls, and calendars packed to the brim push movement to the edges of life, making it something we try to squeeze in rather than live by.

The irony isn't lost on me. I spend much of my time writing, consulting, and researching the science of movement, yet here I am, writing this chapter while sitting at my desk. I make a conscious effort to shift my posture, to stand and stretch, but the reality is that without intention, even those of us who know the science fall into sedentary patterns.

For many people, movement is framed as exercise: a class before work, a run at lunchtime, or a gym session squeezed into the evening. These sessions deliver undeniable benefits for both body and mind but they're not the whole story. Movement doesn't need to be crammed into the margins of your schedule; it's about integrating movement into the rhythm of daily life.

Rethinking movement

Movement is any intentional activity that gets your heart beating, activates your muscles, and increases blood flow to your brain. It's standing up to stretch your legs, twisting in your chair to release that knot between your shoulder blades, it's choosing to walk to the bathroom furthest away from your desk. Even these small movements support both body and mind, improving focus, reducing stress, and lowering long-term health risks.[1]

Movement plays a crucial role in both physical and mental health, from improved cognitive function and regulating stress, to significantly reducing the risk of chronic disease and early mortality.[2] When you move, your brain releases dopamine and serotonin, hormones which not only lift your mood, but also support motivation, energy, and quality sleep. Regular movement also boosts neuroplasticity: your brain's ability to adapt and stay sharp under pressure.

And when you take that movement outside, the benefits multiply. Daylight exposure supports your sleep–wake cycle, while being in nature naturally calms the mind and improves focus. A short walk outdoors isn't just refreshing; it can reset your whole system.

This chapter will explore the science behind movement, debunk common myths, and provide practical strategies to make movement a natural and effortless part of your day. You'll discover how even small bursts of intentional movement can transform your energy, focus, mood, and resilience. You'll also learn why weaving movement into your day, instead of trying to fit it around everything else, is one of the most powerful wellbeing habits you can create.

Meet Matt: Physically active yet drained by the workday

Matt, 37, is climbing fast in the finance sector. His career involves long hours, high-stakes meetings, and never-ending deadlines. He thrives under pressure, priding himself on juggling responsibilities and delivering results, but lately the cost of high performance has started to show.

Despite being diligent about his exercise, hitting the gym at least three evenings a week, Matt feels perpetually drained. His afternoons are marked by sluggish thinking, reduced focus, and an ever-growing dependence on coffee to stay alert. He can't shake the sense that something in his routine is working against him.

At first, he blames his workload. The constant stress, pinging emails, and pressure to perform at the highest level are beginning to take their toll. He tells himself that he just needs to push through, work harder, and find more discipline. But as the weeks turn into months, the exhaustion lingers. He begins zoning out in meetings, snapping at colleagues, and feels mentally spent by mid-afternoon. Even though he's exercising regularly, he doesn't feel physically fit; his body isn't responding the way he expects.

Then, a small yet significant discovery shifts everything. He's recently been gifted a wearable device to track his workouts, and that first evening he notices his step count. What he sees shocks him. Despite his regular gym sessions, and identity as an active person, he's sedentary for nearly ten hours a day. His daily readiness score, a summary of his body's battery, reveals poor recovery from the demands of his workday. Matt realizes he's ticking the exercise box but neglecting the movement his body needs throughout his day.

When we begin working together Matt is determined to make a change. The simplest and most impactful shift is moving his gym sessions from evening to earlier in the day. Intense evening workouts were placing extra strain on an already depleted system, delaying recovery, pushing dinner later, and ultimately disrupting his sleep. By training earlier, his body could recover more effectively, and his evenings became calmer and more restorative.

We also explore adjustments to his work routine. He starts standing for calls, light stretching between tasks, and taking short walks during his lunch break. Instead of relying on coffee to fight his afternoon slump, he energizes with a brisk walk outside. The impact is immediate and powerful. Within weeks he feels sharper, more energetic, and less drained.

By making daytime movement a priority, Matt transforms his workday from one of sedentary exhaustion to one of sustained energy and focus. His story is a powerful reminder that movement isn't just something to schedule beyond the office hours; it's something to build into the rhythm of your workday.

Movement vs exercise: What's the difference?

Movement and exercise are often used interchangeably, but they're not necessarily the same. Exercise is structured, planned, and often goal-oriented; think gym workouts, running, or a yoga session. Movement, on the other hand, is any physical activity that gets you out of prolonged stillness, walking around your home, light stretching between meetings, or standing while on a call. Both are valuable, but movement throughout the day plays a far bigger role in overall health and wellbeing than most people realize.[3]

Movement that powers your day

Imagine having the stamina to tackle high-pressure meetings, demanding deadlines, and personal responsibilities without feeling drained. The key to sustaining this level of performance isn't just mental resilience; it's physical capacity. Just as athletes train their bodies to endure high-intensity competition, you can also use movement to increase your capacity for work and life.

This concept is rooted in the **General Adaptation Syndrome** (GAS), a physiological model explaining how the body adapts to stress.[4] Every activity you do, whether it's physical movement, mental work, or emotional demands, places some level of strain on your body. Even simple, everyday actions create a mild stress response. They deplete your body's battery.

Every time you move, you're not just using energy, you're also expanding your body's capacity to do more. Movement signals your system to adapt, building both physical and mental function over time. In line with the GAS, regular movement strengthens your ability to manage daily demands without tipping into exhaustion. The fitter you are, the more load you can carry, and the less draining everyday tasks become.

Professionals working in high-stress environments, such as surgeons, firefighters, and elite athletes, have long recognized the link between fitness and performance. Maintaining good cardiovascular fitness improves focus, reaction time, and decision-making ability. It's not just about staying in shape; it's about staying sharp, adaptable, and ready to perform when it matters most.

And there's another benefit: consistent movement also supports your immune system. People who exercise regularly are less likely to catch common illnesses like colds and flu. Movement stimulates immune function and reduces inflammation, giving your body another layer of resilience.[5]

For high-achieving professionals like Matt, movement became his competitive advantage. When he started incorporating more movement into his day, he noticed a clear shift in his energy, focus, and ability to manage stress. His workdays felt smoother, and he had more energy left for his personal life. By making movement a habit, you aren't just staying active, you're future proofing your ability to perform at your best.

Reflection moment

Are your daily movement habits charging your body battery or draining it?

How much to move?

For years, you've been told that 150 minutes of moderate-intensity exercise per week (or 75 minutes of vigorous exercise) is the magic number for staying healthy.[6] But if you're like most people, hitting five 30-minute bouts of exercise per week can feel like a challenge.

Every minute of movement counts, and it doesn't need to happen all at once. The more activity you can weave into your daily routine, within your own capacity and limits, the greater the impact on your long-term health, from lowering cardiovascular risk to reducing overall mortality. Imagine what an extra walk, yoga session, or bike ride could mean for your health over time.

Myth busting: The 10,000 steps rule

You've probably heard that 10,000 steps a day is the ideal target for good health, but it's more marketing than science. The number originated from a 1960s Japanese pedometer slogan, not from rigorous research. What matters more is progress. If you're not near 10,000 steps per day, start by adding 1,000 extra steps per week. Small, manageable increases in movement compound over time, delivering powerful long-term benefits without adding extra strain to your schedule. It's not just about the number of steps you take; it's about how you move and how consistently you weave movement into your day.

The hidden cost of sitting

Many people believe that hitting the gym three times a week or exercising 30 minutes a day is enough to counteract hours of sitting, yet prolonged sitting of more than eight hours per day still increases the risk of cardiovascular disease, Type 2 diabetes, and musculoskeletal problems, even when you exercise regularly.

Excessive sitting is now considered the new smoking in terms of health risks. It leads to reduced oxygen flow to the brain, slowing cognitive performance and increasing feelings of sluggishness.[7] A cruel reminder that your evening exercise class or trip to the gym is not enough to counteract what happens between workouts.

Prolonged sitting leads to neck and back pain which aren't just inconveniences. Musculoskeletal conditions drive substantial productivity loss across sectors, and in many organizations, sit alongside mental health as a top driver for long-term absence.[8]

The productivity paradox

Many of us kid ourselves into thinking that staying seated and focused for extended periods leads to higher productivity, but don't be fooled. Tools and systems designed to streamline workflow can contribute to cognitive overload. Endless updates, distractions, and notifications fragment attention and blunt efficiency.

Sitting more does not equate to getting more work done. Working longer and harder often leads to diminishing returns and raises health risks; the World Health Organization links working 55 hours or more per week with a 35% higher risk of stroke than working 35–40 hours.[9] Brief movement breaks, such as light stretching, walking, or standing desk work, help regulate cortisol, reset cognitive function and improve productivity.[10] For Matt, a simple habit of standing for phone calls and taking short walking breaks each afternoon, shifted his post-lunch clarity and performance.

The role of posture in preventing fatigue

Posture refers to the way you hold your body when sitting, standing, or moving. It's more than just how you look; it plays a critical role in how you feel and function. Supportive posture aligns the spine, reduces strain on muscles and joints, and promotes overall physical wellbeing. Conversely, poor posture can lead to discomfort, fatigue, and long-term health issues. Simple strategies, such as dynamic sitting, can help prevent stiffness and discomfort.

Dynamic sitting involves engaging different muscle groups while seated by making small, intentional movements such as adjusting posture, shifting weight, or performing subtle seated exercises. These exercises include seated pelvic tilts, shoulder rolls, and hand press, all of which help maintain engagement of postural muscles while reducing strain from prolonged sitting.[11] Practising these movements for just a couple of minutes every 45 to 60 minutes reduces stiffness, improves circulation, and supports spinal health.

Even when you consider the rise of standing desks, walking meetings, and parking a distance from the office, most people still spend the majority of the workday sitting. You don't need to stand all day, you need variety, frequent micro-breaks and postural shifts that support your core and keep you alert.

Protect your posture

- ✓ **Avoid common stressors**: slumping, crossing your legs, or leaning to one side strains your spine and neck, compresses breathing, and leads to fatigue and discomfort.
- ✓ **Posture goals**: aim for an active, supportive posture. Sit tall through your hips, feet flat, light core engagement, shoulders relaxed and your screen at eye level.
- ✓ **Small adjustments**: every 45–60 minutes, stand, roll your shoulders, do ten calf raises, or take a 2–3-minute corridor walk. Standing all day isn't the answer, regular movement is. Think of these as movement snacks for your overall wellbeing.

Even small daily adjustments can create a meaningful difference in overall wellbeing. Matt's experience echoed this. His afternoon energy dips, difficulty concentrating, and sense of tiredness were exacerbated by excessive sitting. He soon realized that he couldn't rely on his evening workouts; he needed to integrate movement during his workday.

Regular movement not only boosts overall wellbeing, it protects musculoskeletal health. High levels of sedentary behaviour at work are strongly associated with increased reports of back and neck pain, leading to diminished productivity.[12] Building simple postural adjustments into your day can ease muscle tension, support spinal alignment, and prevent common workplace-related pain.

The science of small movements

It's easy to think fitness is built only in the gym, but the truth is that *the way* you move in everyday life matters just as much and sometimes more. Scientists call this **Non-Exercise Activity Thermogenesis** (NEAT). These are the small, often unnoticed movements, like pacing on a call, tidying your desk, or walking to the furthest bathroom, that steadily add up to make a big difference.

People with higher NEAT levels burn significantly more calories per day than those who are sedentary, even if they exercise regularly.[13] In fact, one of the reasons why some people gain weight more easily than others isn't necessarily due to differences in workout routines but in these small, daily movements they make outside of exercise.

The benefits don't stop at burning calories. NEAT also supports mental clarity, focus, and emotional regulation. For those in desk-based roles, this is particularly important. One burst of exercise can't undo 10 hours of sitting, but small, consistent movements can make a real difference.

When Matt started incorporating these tiny movements into his day, instead of forcing movement into rigid exercise blocks, he moved more often. By reframing movement as an ongoing part of his day, rather than something requiring extra time, he significantly boosted his energy levels and focus. NEAT is the secret weapon for health and performance. You don't need to overhaul your routine, just move a little more, a little more often. Balance ball instead of an office-chair anyone?

Movement that resets stress

Movement is more than just a way to stay active; it is a powerful way to regulate stress and optimize brain performance. As you explored in the previous chapter, persistently elevated cortisol, the body's primary stress hormone, can disrupt sleep, drain energy, and undermine wellbeing. Physical activity helps lower cortisol levels and acts as a reset button, reducing stress accumulation before it takes a toll on your mental and physical health.

Matt's story illustrates this well. Before he incorporated movement into his day, his body was in a near-constant state of stress shown through sustained high resting heart rate (RHR) and low daily readiness scores. His body struggled to recover. But after adding regular movements, such as walking between tasks, his stress levels began to stabilize. He not only felt more energized, but he also slept better, focused more easily, and handled pressure with greater ease. The connection between movement, sleep, and sustained energy is profound. Movement doesn't just lower stress; it creates a ripple effect that improves both mental and physical capacity.

Reflection moment

When stress builds, what's one simple movement you could do right now to reset, a walk, a stretch, or a deep breath, before you dive into the next task?

As you aim to increase your daily movement, it's important to remember that more isn't always better. Pushing activity levels too far, even with good intentions, can start to work against your health and performance. Let's take a closer look at how training beyond your capacity can erode the very gains you're working so hard to achieve.

When more isn't always better

There's a growing trend of professionals turning to high-intensity exercise to 'burn-off' work stress, often pushing their bodies to the limit.[14] While regular exercise is beneficial, too much of a good thing can backfire because the body doesn't differentiate between physical, mental, and emotional stress.

Whether it's stress on your body from a tough workout, a packed schedule, or emotional overwhelm, *all* forms of stress load your body's systems. Without sufficient recovery, even healthy habits like exercise can start tipping into depletion. That's when movement stops building capacity and starts draining energy, disrupting sleep, and increasing the risk of burnout.

For high performers who thrive on structure and pushing limits, it can be tempting to think that more is always better, but excessive high-intensity training without adequate recovery can elevate stress hormones like cortisol, leading to the same physiological strain as chronic workplace burnout. The goal isn't to do more; it's to balance stress and recovery, ensuring exercise builds capacity rather than drains it.

Prioritizing recovery through sleep, active rest days, and lower-intensity movement like walking or yoga ensures that training remains beneficial rather than detrimental. Recognizing the importance of movement is just the first step. The next is personalizing it. This is where wearable technology helps you match effort with recovery in real time, allowing you to adapt to the day you're actually having, not the one you pencilled in.

What your wearable tells you about Your Movement Habit

When lives are busy, with desk-bound, sedentary jobs, it's easy to misjudge how much (or how little) you move. You overestimate your activity and underestimate your need for recovery. That's where wearable technology changes the game.

Wearables do more than just count steps. Some use movement rings or daily activity *scores*, while others focus on **strain**, **readiness**, or **training load**. They give you real-time, personalized feedback on your movement patterns, energy levels, and recovery needs, helping you spot movement trends you might otherwise miss. They hold up a mirror to your habits, offering insights that empower you to move with more intention, balance, and impact.

Resting heart rate

As your fitness improves through regular movement, your heart will become more efficient, and your RHR may gradually lower. This is your body's way of telling you it's adapting. On days when your RHR is unusually high, it may signal stress, fatigue, or that your body needs recovery.

What to look for:

- Check your RHR while still lying down in bed and over time you'll become familiar with your average.
- If you notice an elevated RHR in the morning, relative to the day before, this suggests that your system is struggling to recover from previous workouts or daily stressors; use it as a cue to prioritize gentle movement or active recovery.

Step count and activity monitoring

Step counts can be useful, but they don't differentiate between meaningful movement and low-intensity activity. Many wearables will capture much more than how many steps you take; they track how frequently you move, how long you stay inactive, and whether your activity is truly benefiting your body.

Remember 10,000 steps is not the gold standard you were led to believe. A single walk may help you hit your step goal, but if you remain sedentary for the rest of the day, the benefits are significantly reduced. Wearable data can highlight when you've been inactive for too long and help you break the cycle of prolonged sitting.

Instead of fixating on a target number, use your step count to notice trends and find small opportunities to move more. Whether it's taking a walking call, stretching between meetings, or getting outside for a brisk walk, every step counts. Moving more isn't about meeting a quota; it's about building momentum.

What to look for:

- What is your daily target? How does your target align with your fitness goals? Remember even modest increases can benefit health.
- Have you noticed any sudden reduction in step count? These can indicate busy, screen-heavy days that would benefit from a short walk or quick stretch.
- Does your wearable let you know how many active minutes you have per day? Track time spent in moderate to vigorous activity to ensure you're meeting recommended exercise guidelines.
- Have you turned your notifications on for movement alerts? If you ignore movement alerts, you're not just missing an opportunity to stretch, you're allowing stress and fatigue to build up, negating some of the benefits of your workouts and making you feel more depleted as the day goes on.

Training load

Many wearables also calculate your training load, or *strain*, a measure of how much physical stress your body is carrying, by combining several key metrics. These typically include average and peak heart rate, exercise duration and intensity, plus recovery metrics when available. Training load offers a clear picture of how demanding your recent activity has been on your cardiovascular system, muscles, and overall recovery capacity.

What to look for:

- Look for trends in your scores. If your training load gradually increases in a sustainable way, it's a sign that you're building fitness.
- Aim for balanced loading. This will be seen through a mix of high strain days with easier, recovery-focused days.

Heart rate variability

Monitoring your heart rate variability (HRV) provides valuable insights into how well your body is adapting to changes in demand and stress. And let's not forget that exercising causes a strain on your body. By regularly exercising you build up your fitness levels and your body will cope with greater demands. With consistent training, many people see their HRV rise over time, a sign their body is coping more effectively with stress.

What to look for:

- A high HRV generally suggests that your nervous system is adaptable, switching efficiently between the effort of exercise and recovery. Your body is responding well to movement, stress, and daily demands.
- If you notice a trend over time of your HRV remaining low after an intense workout or a period of high stress, your body may be telling you to prioritize rest. Instead

of pushing harder, incorporate active recovery, such as walking, stretching, or yoga, to help restore balance and prevent long-term fatigue.

- A key indicator that you might be training beyond your capacity is a consistently lower than usual HRV score, even when you're getting enough sleep. This suggests your nervous system is staying in a heightened stress state rather than shifting into recovery mode.

Sleep duration and quality insights

Sleep and movement are deeply connected, each one influencing the other. Daytime activity helps you fall asleep more easily and recover more deeply, while restorative sleep gives you the energy to stay active the following day.

What to look for:

- Is your sleep improving with consistent movement throughout your day?
- Are you short on deep sleep? Light daytime activity often improves sleep quality, which in turn supports better motivation, energy, and emotional resilience, making it easier to stay active the next day.
- Is evening exercise disrupting your sleep quality or sleep latency (how long it takes to fall asleep)? You might need to reschedule moderate to high-intensity exercise to before work or earlier in the evening.

Reflection moment

What's one small change to your movement habit that would support better sleep tonight?

Daily readiness score

Visualize your capacity for movement as an energy gauge, just like the fuel gauge in a car. On many wearables it's presented as your readiness score or **body battery**. The score combines data from your RHR, HRV, sleep quality, and recent activity to give you a real-time snapshot of how well recovered your body is to move.

What to look for:

- If your body readiness score is low (typically under 40), lighter movement is better for your wellbeing and regaining balance. Choose activities that won't drain your energy such as a mindful walk or gentle yoga stretches.
- If your body readiness score is high (typically 80–100) this is your signal that you are ready for more intensity. Your battery is charged. This is the ideal time for more intense movement and workouts focused on strength and fitness. You're in the exercise zone and you're ready to go.
- If your readiness score is too low, you've drained your battery; it's when the warning light comes on. Any intense exercise within this low score zone would put too great a strain on your body, leading to excessive strain, fatigue, or even burnout.

Reflection moment

If you're planning a training session after a stressful day, pause to ask:

Will the session energize you or add more stress?

Could something gentler, like a brisk walk or yoga, leave you more refreshed tomorrow?

While your wearable provides real-time feedback on movement gaps, step count, and energy patterns, it's only part of the story. Tuning into how you *feel* while moving offers insight that data alone can't capture.

Your movement breakthrough

Tuning into your body's natural rhythm is the key to building a movement habit that feels good, fits your life, and fuels your wellbeing, not just now, but long term. True transformation comes from reflecting on the story behind the numbers using the 'Aha Model' of awareness, habit, action. The following questions are designed to help uncover your movement patterns, identify potential gaps, and reframe daily movement as a conscious choice rather than a reactive habit.

Awareness: Identifying your movement gaps

Before adding more movement to your routine, it's important to first identify where the gaps are. Wearable data can help, but you don't need technology to build movement awareness. Begin by observing your own activity patterns to spot where small changes can be made. Spend three–five days paying attention to your daily activity. You won't need detailed notes, just brief observations. Consider:

- *How many hours did you spend sitting today?*
- *When during the day were you most inactive (e.g. mornings, long meetings, evenings)?*
- *Were there natural pauses when you could have moved but didn't?*
- *Did you notice stiffness, fatigue, or restlessness at any point?*
- *How many short movement breaks did you take?*
- *Did you include any intentional movement (e.g. a walk, yoga, light stretching)?*

Most people find there are parts of the day that are consistently sedentary and even small gaps in their day cumulate to long periods of stillness. By identifying your personal movement gaps, you lay the foundation for designing habits that work with your day, not against it.

Reflection moment

What would a perfect day of movement look like for you?

How would achieving greater movement impact the rest of your day/week?

What obstacles have prevented you from moving more, and how can you overcome them?

Habit: Embedding movement into your daily routine

Now that you've spotted when movement is missing in your day, it's time to choose the habit you want to build into your routine. You might decide to schedule something structured, like a run before work, a regular lunchtime walk, or an exercise class after work. These activities can be planned and scheduled in advance. But to keep your body moving throughout the workday itself, start by identifying a movement habit that you can integrate into your daily routine.

Behavioural scientist Susan Michie and colleagues provide a useful framework for choosing your habit: **the COM-B model**. It shows that capability, opportunity, and motivation combine to make behaviour change possible.[15] When choosing your movement habit consider:

- ***Capability**: Can you do this safely and consistently with your current fitness and skills?*
- ***Opportunity**: Where does this naturally fit into your day and environment and do you have the kit, space, and support?*
- ***Motivation**: Does it feel rewarding or meaningful to you, and what small cue will keep you coming back?*

When all of these are in place, your habit has a strong chance of sticking.

Action: Reinforcing movement to make it stick

Have you ever set an intention to exercise more, only to find yourself skipping it because it felt like too much effort? You're not the only one!

It's not unusual to set an intention to build a new habit only to find it neglected after the first week.

Shawn Achor offers a practical solution to this challenge with his **20-second rule**; a strategy to make it easier to build good habits and harder to maintain unhelpful ones.[16] The science behind it is simple. The more friction, effort, decision-making, or resistance involved in starting a habit, the less likely you are to follow through. Your brain naturally seeks the path of least resistance, preferring what is easiest and most convenient.

If movement feels complicated, your brain will choose the easier option: staying put. But if you can reduce the friction, you're more likely to follow through. For example, if your gym kit and trainers are buried in a drawer, you're far less likely to exercise than if you get them out the night before. That 20-second difference can make or break your consistency. You don't need specialist equipment or a perfect plan to get started. Simply standing, stretching, or walking is enough. The easier it is to start moving, ideally within 20 seconds, the more likely you are to build the habit.

Many people wait to feel motivated before they act, but Achor's research shows it's the other way around: action triggers motivation. Once you take the first small step, momentum builds, and the motivation to continue often follows. This is especially important for busy professionals who struggle to integrate movement into their day, the key is to start small, start quickly, and let momentum do the rest.

Move in 20 seconds

✓ **Prepare in advance**: lay out comfortable shoes, keep a resistance band near your desk, or have a stretching area set up. When movement is easy to access, you're more likely to do it.

- ✓ **Reduce the steps to start**: if getting outside feels like too much effort, start with two minutes of movement indoors. Once you've started, you'll often keep going.
- ✓ **Use visual reminders**: a sticky note that says 'stand up' or an alert on your smartwatch makes movement an automatic prompt rather than a forced decision.
- ✓ **Pair movement with existing habits**: attach movement to something you already do, stand while checking emails, stretch after meetings, or do calf raises while brushing your teeth.
- ✓ **Remove friction for good habits**: if sitting all day is the default, adjust your workspace so standing is easier.

At first, Matt found it difficult to break the habit of sitting for hours at his desk. Even though he wanted to move more, the activation energy required to stand up, decide what movement to do, and actually do it, felt like a barrier.

This 20-second rule was key for Matt. He often told himself he'd take a movement break later, when he had 'more time' or 'felt like it'. But later never came. To fix this, he created a path of least resistance; he set an alarm to stand up every 45 minutes, no decision-making required.

Before long, through consistency and patience, movement stopped feeling like an effort and started feeling natural. Over time, these micro-habits became part of his daily routine, boosting his mood, focus, and energy. Remember, the easier movement is to start, the harder it becomes to ignore.

Reflection moment

What's one simple shift you could make today to remove friction and move more easily?

Don't forget to acknowledge your progress. Pause to notice how movement lifts your focus and mood, or how a lunchtime walk boosts your afternoon energy and evening resilience. Take a moment and check in: *How do you feel?*

For movement to become a natural part of your day, positive reinforcement and small wins matter. The more you connect movement with enjoyment and success, the more likely it is to feel automatic, satisfying, and worth repeating. By using self-reflection you can move beyond passive tracking and start making intentional choices that enhance your movement advantage. Remember, small shifts, practised consistently, lead to big results.

Your move towards better wellbeing

Movement is not an optional extra, it's a core pillar of your wellbeing advantage. The human body has evolved to function best when in motion, yet modern lifestyles have stripped movement from our daily routines, leading to prolonged periods of sedentary behaviour, which is far from ideal.

How you move throughout your day impacts everything, from your energy levels and stress resilience to cognitive function and long-term health. And as you've seen, it's not just about scheduled workouts and bouts of exercise before and after work. The science is clear: it's about weaving movement seamlessly into your daily routine, making it as natural as breathing.

Matt's story demonstrates how structured exercise cannot compensate for an otherwise sedentary lifestyle. His reliance on three weekly workouts gave him a false sense of movement adequacy, while his wearable data revealed the physiological strain caused by prolonged sitting. By making small but intentional movement shifts throughout the day, standing, stretching, walking between meetings, he significantly improved his energy, cognitive performance, and overall wellbeing, all without adding a single extra workout.

And this is your opportunity too. Your body is built for movement, and the more you align with that natural design, the better you'll feel. The key is consistency over intensity, moving more often, not just more strenuously. The best movement habit is the one you can stick with. Whether it's a break to stretch, a short walk, or adjusting your posture, each movement counts toward building a stronger, more energized version of yourself. Simply put, frequent low-intensity movement is vital in supporting sustained energy, cognitive sharpness, and stress resilience.

Movement is just one piece of the puzzle. What fuels your body is just as important as how you move it. In the next chapter, you'll explore how to nourish your body in a way that supports your movement habits, sustains energy levels, and enhances recovery, helping you not just move more but thrive more.

Let's unlock the next part of your wellbeing toolkit, fuelling your body for sustained energy, focus, and resilience.

Boost your movement

- ✓ **Set a reminder**: stretch or stand every 45 minutes to reset posture and blood flow.
- ✓ **Insert micro-breaks**: take a 2-minute movement break between tasks to clear mental fog.
- ✓ **Use body-weight moves**: add squats, calf raises, and wall sits to re-energize quickly.
- ✓ **Choose the stairs when possible**: short climbs lift heart rate and counter sitting spells.
- ✓ **Suggest active meetings**: try walking meetings or stand-up discussions to keep energy up.
- ✓ **Add seated mobility**: do ankle circles, spinal twists, and shoulder rolls to ease tension.

3

Your Nutrition Habit

Think for a moment about how you treat your phone, your laptop, even your car. You charge them, update them, fuel them with the best, to keep them performing at their best. But when it comes to the most sophisticated system you own, your body and mind, are you fuelling them with the same level of care?

When life gets hectic, it's easy for poor eating habits to take hold. Meals get skipped, sweet snacks become your quick fix and coffee fills the gaps. The cost is high. Fast-digesting carbohydrate and sugary treats cause blood sugar spikes, followed by crashes that drain focus and trigger mood swings. This energy rollercoaster is a leading cause of burnout in busy professionals.[1]

The good news is you don't need a perfect diet or a complicated meal plan. With just a few simple shifts, you can start nourishing yourself in a way that supports your wellbeing throughout the day, not just at mealtimes.

Nutrition as your competitive advantage

Nutrition has traditionally been viewed through the lens of physical health: energy, weight, and fitness. Yet we're now beginning to recognize its untapped potential as a performance tool for the mind. In the same way that you recharge your batteries overnight, the nutrients you consume throughout the day determine how resilient you feel under pressure, how alert you remain in long meetings, and how calm you stay when faced with unexpected demands. And here's the truth: if you're not fuelling your body well, you're throwing stress into overdrive, leaving yourself more reactive, less focused, and increasingly drained.

Shift your mindset from eating to get through the day to eating to perform at your best, and nutrition becomes a powerful advantage. When you treat your eating habits as opportunities to build resilience, enhance focus, and support emotional stability it allows you to build capacity and sharpen your edge.

This chapter is not about weight management, specialist diets, or clinical conditions. Instead, it invites you to reframe nutrition as part of your wellbeing toolkit. Rather than prescribing a rigid plan, we'll focus on a balanced, flexible approach that fits the realities of a busy life. Many of the principles you'll find here, prioritizing whole foods, healthy fats, and slow-digesting carbohydrates, are reflected in healthy eating plans like the Mediterranean diet.[2] With its emphasis on vegetables, wholegrains, oily fish, and extra-virgin olive oil, this style of eating offers a foundation for long-term health and performance while complementing the strategies you'll explore in this chapter.

You'll discover how food and hydration aren't just tools for maintaining physical health; they help sustain your energy, elevate mood, and provide a buffer against the stressors of modern life. You'll also find proven behaviour change models ensuring the changes you make aren't short-term fixes but lifelong, sustainable habits that will become part of your day-to-day routine.

Let's start by uncovering the powerful connection between nutrition and productivity through the journey of Nick. Like many busy professionals, he relied on caffeine and convenience foods to get through the day, only to find his energy crashing and focus fading. By making a few simple yet impactful changes to his eating and hydrating habits, Nick shifted from low energy, mood swings, and reliance on quick fixes to a steadier, more sustainable rhythm. His story offers valuable lessons that can inspire your own transformation.

Meet Nick: Fuelled by caffeine and convenience

Nick, 39, is a senior project manager, navigating back-to-back meetings across time zones. His days are driven by urgency: tight deadlines, rapid decision-making, and the relentless pressure to deliver high-performance results.

His mornings are a mad dash, racing to catch the early train, often running on empty. Breakfast, if any, is a quick coffee and pastry grabbed from the station kiosk. Coffee isn't a treat, it's his lifeline. Not just one or two cups, but up to eight a day, fuelling a cycle of artificial alertness and deeper fatigue.

Lunch is rarely planned, usually whatever he can grab quickly between calls, if he remembers at all. Some days it's a sandwich, other days just a coffee. The mid-afternoon crash comes like clockwork: brain fog, sugar cravings, and low motivation. He'll grab crisps or a chocolate bar for a boost, hoping to power through. Come evening, his unwind ritual includes a couple of beers, screen time, and a restless night's sleep.

Nick has normalized this routine. But his body hasn't. When persistent low energy, irritability, and poor sleep start to interfere with both his work and home life, Nick knows something needs to change. His wearable data backs up what he's feeling: his heart rate variability (HRV) (a marker of recovery capacity) is consistently lower than his usual baseline, overnight recovery is poor, and his resting heart rate (RHR) hovers too high. His body is stuck in stress mode.

As part of a broader wellbeing programme, we focus on small, sustainable nutritional changes rather than a complete overhaul. First, he introduces a protein-rich breakfast: eggs with wholegrain toast or granola paired with Greek yogurt, to help stabilize his blood sugar and sustain energy. Gradually, he reduces his reliance on coffee by choosing decaffeinated options and using hydration reminders to drink more water. For lunch he switches from plain sandwiches to wholegrain chicken salad wraps and fruit to increase protein and fibre. In the evening, he replaces his mid-week beer with an alcohol-free version and begins winding down earlier.

These tweaks may seem minor, but within weeks, Nick feels the difference. Afternoon slumps ease, his focus sharpens, and his mood evens out. His wearable reflects the shift too, with higher daily readiness scores, improved sleep quality, and recovery indicators such as steadier RHR and better HRV trends.

If you've ever felt stuck in a cycle of low energy, food cravings, or stress, Nick's story is your reminder: change doesn't require a complete reset. It starts with one habit, one choice, one shift. Nick's transformation isn't about perfection. It's about being intentional. Nutritionally, he comes to understand that it's not about getting every meal right. A slice of cake or a takeaway now and then? Absolutely. Food should nourish and bring joy; it's about your pattern of nutrition across the week.

Nutrition powers performance

Balanced nutrition is more than the sum of calories; it's the quality of what you consume and the consistency with which you consume it. At its core, a balanced diet includes a variety of whole foods, proteins, complex carbohydrates (including wholegrains and vegetables), healthy fats, vitamins, minerals, and water, that work in harmony to support the body and brain.

When these elements are out of balance, when you lean on heavily processed carbohydrates, skip meals, or rely on caffeine and sugar, the body responds by triggering a stress cascade. Blood sugar fluctuates. Energy crashes. Irritability spikes. Concentration wavers. Over time, this invisible nutritional imbalance compounds, undermining your performance and wellbeing.[3]

Reflection moment

In what ways are your food choices affecting how you show up each day, at work and beyond?

The energy rollercoaster

You've likely felt it, the post-pastry high followed by the mid-afternoon slump where focus fades and patience wears thin. You reach for a snack or another coffee, and the cycle repeats. The **energy rollercoaster** driven by blood sugar instability, is one of the most overlooked contributors to burnout, especially in high-performing professionals who are already running on empty.[4] Let's explore what's happening beneath the surface.

When you eat foods high in refined carbohydrates and sugars, such as white bread, pastries, sugary cereals, biscuits, or sweetened drinks, glucose enters the bloodstream rapidly, triggering a sharp rise in blood sugar (otherwise known as a glucose spike). You feel a temporary lift in energy, clarity, and mood.

In response, your pancreas releases insulin to shuttle that glucose into your cells for energy. But with high-sugar meals and snacks, the insulin response often overshoots, leading to a rapid dip in blood sugar levels. This dip is the crash, the afternoon slump you're all too aware of.

Low blood sugar then triggers the release of cortisol, your body's primary stress hormone, to restore balance by prompting more energy-seeking behaviour, hence the craving for caffeine or another sugary fix. The rollercoaster ride continues.

With the crash comes more than just fatigue. You may feel foggy, irritable, unmotivated, and desperate for something sweet or caffeinated to get you through the next task. Over time, these fluctuations keep your nervous system in 'fight-or-flight' mode, gradually depleting your resilience and making stress harder to regulate. This isn't weakness; it's your body reacting to unstable fuel.

Break the cycle with smarter fuel

One of the simplest and most effective strategies for avoiding the rollercoaster is to include adequate protein in every meal and snack. Protein slows digestion, which prevents rapid spikes and dips in blood sugar. It also provides the building blocks for important brain chemicals like dopamine and serotonin. These are the neurotransmitters that help you stay motivated, emotionally balanced, and mentally resilient when things get tough at work.

By understanding how blood sugar affects stress and stamina, you can start fuelling in a way that supports, not sabotages, your performance. Your energy doesn't need to come in bursts. It can be steady, sustainable, and satisfying with just a few simple, strategic changes.

Small swaps, more protein

- ✓ **Breakfast**: add Greek yogurt to your oats. Swap jam for nut butter.
- ✓ **Lunch**: top salads with grilled chicken, salmon, tofu, or chickpeas.
- ✓ **Dinner**: mix black beans or lentils into your casseroles and curries.
- ✓ **Snacks**: try carrot sticks and hummus, mixed nuts, or boiled eggs.

The gut–brain connection

You've probably heard the phrase *trust your gut*. But your gut does more than send instinctive nudges, it actively shapes how you think, feel, and cope with stress.

Science now confirms what many have suspected for years: your gut is directly connected to your brain. This relationship, known as the **gut–brain axis**, is a complex two-way communication system between your digestive system and central nervous system. It's why your gut health can influence everything from mood and immunity to focus and resilience.

In fact, your gut produces around 90% of your body's serotonin, a key neurotransmitter that regulates mood, sleep, and emotional balance. The health of your gut microbiome, the trillions of bacteria and microbes that live in your digestive tract, has been shown to affect how much of this *feel-good* chemical your body can produce and regulate.

Feel-good foods to support the gut–brain axis

- ✓ **Fibre-rich foods**: oats, whole grains, lentils, beans, chickpeas, apples, and pears.
- ✓ **Fermented foods**: live yogurt, kefir, kimchi, sauerkraut, miso.
- ✓ **Omega-3 sources**: salmon, mackerel, sardines, flaxseeds, chia seeds, walnuts.
- ✓ **Prebiotic-rich foods**: garlic, onions, leeks, asparagus, bananas.
- ✓ **Polyphenol-rich foods**: blueberries, dark chocolate (70%+), green tea, olive oil.

Your immune system starts in the gut

Around 70% of your immune system is associated with the gut, making it one of the most important defenders of your health. That's because your gut lining is home to a vast community of microbes that constantly interact with your immune cells. Tim Spector, professor of genetic epidemiology and a leading authority on gut health, explains that when your digestive system is healthy, the gut–brain connection helps you stay resilient, both physically and mentally.[5] But when gut health is sub-optimal whether from stress, a poor diet, or overuse of antibiotics, it can weaken immune defences, trigger low-grade inflammation and make it harder to bounce back from physical and mental strain.

For professionals under constant pressure, this matters more than you might think. Chronic stress already challenges your immune system; add in gut imbalance, and you may find yourself more prone to illness, slower to recover from intense work periods, or feeling constantly drained. If you're constantly feeling run down, foggy or flat, even after a full night's sleep, your gut might be part of the picture.

The hidden cost of processed food

Processed foods, especially those high in refined sugar and trans fats, can trigger systemic inflammation that affects not only your body but also your brain function. Chris van Tulleken, an infectious-disease doctor and one of the UK's most vocal critics of ultra-processed foods, explains how these highly engineered products disrupt appetite, mood regulation, and resilience, making it harder for professionals to sustain energy and focus under pressure.[6] This happens because inflammatory cytokines (chemical messengers released by immune cells) can interfere with brain function, reduce neuroplasticity (your brain's ability to adapt and stay sharp under pressure), and make your stress response more reactive and harder to regulate.

By contrast, when you regularly nourish your body with brain-supportive foods, like oily fish, leafy greens, nuts, berries, and wholegrains, you're giving your brain what it needs to perform at its best. You're more likely to feel alert, focused, and resilient. You may notice yourself thinking more clearly, solving problems more easily, and responding to challenges with greater calm. This is the power of high-performance nutrition.

Brain boosting nutrition

- ✓ **Oily fish**: salmon, mackerel, sardines, trout.
- ✓ **Leafy greens**: spinach, kale, rocket, Swiss chard, broccoli.
- ✓ **Berries**: blueberries, strawberries, blackberries, raspberries.
- ✓ **Wholegrains**: oats, quinoa, brown rice, barley, wholegrain bread.
- ✓ **Nuts and seeds**: walnuts, flaxseeds, chia seeds, pumpkin seeds, almonds.
- ✓ **Legumes**: lentils, chickpeas, black beans (rich in fibre and B vitamins).
- ✓ **Healthy fats**: extra-virgin olive oil, avocado.

The most overlooked performance tool

Water might not be the first thing you think of when considering your wellbeing, performance or mental clarity, but it should be. Hydration is one of the simplest and most effective ways to support energy, focus, and emotional regulation. Yet, it's also one of the most neglected.

Hydration supports your nervous system by regulating stress responses, maintaining emotional balance, and enhancing cognitive clarity. When you're well-hydrated, you think faster, respond more effectively under pressure, and feel more alert and less depleted as the day progresses.[7] Staying hydrated is more than a simple health tip; it's a foundation for sustained mental performance and resilience.

When the body is dehydrated, cortisol, the primary stress hormone, tends to rise. Even mild dehydration could mean losing your edge in a meeting, struggling to focus on a task, or becoming more reactive in a difficult conversation. If any of this feels familiar, it may not be stress or lack of sleep, it could be that your body and brain are under-hydrated.

Many professionals remain chronically dehydrated, due to excessive caffeine, long stretches without water, or forgetting to drink throughout the day. Most people wait until they feel thirsty before drinking, but thirst is a late-stage signal; by the time it shows up you're already on the way to dehydration. Keeping a fresh water bottle close by can make a big difference.

Silent signs of dehydration

- ✓ Afternoon fatigue.
- ✓ Irritability or mood dips.
- ✓ Brain fog or forgetfulness.
- ✓ Headaches.
- ✓ Difficulty focusing.

A strong coffee to start the day. A glass of wine to wind down at night. For many of us this routine feels normal, even necessary. But when overused or mistimed they can erode energy, interfere with stress recovery, and significantly reduce the quality of your sleep.

The caffeine trap: Alert now, tired later

Let's start with caffeine. While it can enhance alertness and concentration in the short term, caffeine works by blocking **adenosine**, a chemical in the brain that builds up throughout the day to signal sleepiness. Blocking it gives you that 'awake' feeling. But the more caffeine you consume, and the later in the day you consume it, the more you disrupt your body's natural rhythms.

A word of caution: your caffeine can stay in your system for up to 8–10 hours which means your 3 p.m. coffee may still be interfering with your sleep at 11 p.m. Matthew Walker, Professor of Neuroscience and Psychology at the University of California, Berkeley and founder of the Center for Human Sleep Science, reminds us that even if you fall asleep easily, caffeine reduces the amount of deep, restorative sleep you get, meaning you wake up less refreshed, less focused, and more reliant on stimulants the next day.[8]

Caffeine is also a diuretic, which means it increases the need to urinate. While this might seem minor, for office workers tied to back-to-back meetings or reliant on maintaining blocks of focus at their desk, it can create ongoing interruptions and contribute to dehydration. Dehydration, in turn, affects concentration, increases fatigue, and can trigger headaches or mood dips, none of which are conducive to a productive workday.

If you find yourself making extra trips to the loo after your third coffee or feeling parched by midday, it's worth considering whether caffeine could be contributing more stress than support. It's never too late to check out the decaffeinated alternatives for your afternoon coffee break.

The sleep disruptor hiding in your evening routine

Then there's alcohol. While it may help you relax initially, alcohol disrupts the architecture of your sleep. Many people have a complex relationship with alcohol; it's often social, habitual, or a way to self-soothe after a long day. This book isn't about judging those choices or exploring the deeper issues surrounding alcohol dependence, instead, the focus is on understanding the very real and measurable ways alcohol affects your wellbeing and performance.

Even small amounts of alcohol can impact your recovery, emotional regulation, and ability to handle the demands of work and life. Alcohol also impacts blood sugar regulation and cortisol levels, both of which play key roles in how energized and stable you feel the following day. What feels like a temporary stress-reliever often creates a bigger stress load on the body.

In my work using wearable technology to track lifestyle patterns, the most consistent and damaging effects of alcohol are seen in its disruption of sleep and recovery. For many of my clients, even small amounts of alcohol lead to fragmented sleep, reducing the brain's ability to consolidate memory, regulate emotions, and recharge overnight. As a result, they wake feeling exhausted, emotionally reactive, and weighed down by challenges that would normally feel manageable. Over time, this cycle contributes to mounting fatigue, reduced resilience, and a growing sense of burnout at work.

Nick discovered this first hand. His evening routine of just a couple of beers never felt excessive. It was, after all, his way of switching off. But combined with several cups of coffee during his demanding workday, the impact on his sleep and recovery was undeniable. His wearable device showed he was getting around six hours of sleep each night, but only two hours of that was classified as restorative sleep. In short, he was getting sleep, but not the kind his body and brain needed to recharge.

Sleep-safe choices for caffeine and alcohol

- ✓ **Time caffeine wisely**: keep caffeine to the first half of the day (ideally before 2 p.m.) to protect your natural sleep drive and overnight recovery.
- ✓ **Alternate your coffees**: swap every other coffee for a non-caffeinated drink (water, herbal tea) to reduce total intake without losing the ritual.
- ✓ **Plan alcohol-free days**: build in regular alcohol-free days to improve sleep quality and next-day energy.
- ✓ **Switch it up**: on evenings out switch to non-alcoholic options after your first drink to support restorative sleep.

Building your nutrition advantage

When it comes to any change in your lifestyle, consistency is better than perfection. Even with the best of intentions, the reality of a busy, high-pressure job can easily derail healthy eating habits. Whether it's stress-eating during a tough day, grabbing whatever's convenient when time is tight, or struggling with long-term weight concerns, many professionals face similar hurdles. Let's explore some of the most common challenges to building your nutrition advantage and practical strategies to navigate them.

It's easy to blame yourself for a lack of willpower when you reach for chocolate instead of fruit or skip lunch only to binge on snacks later. But the truth is, willpower is a limited resource. When you're tired, overworked, or emotionally drained, your brain will default to whatever is easiest and most comforting. This isn't weakness; it's biology. The key is not to rely on willpower alone, but to design your environment so that better choices become easier to make.

Reflection moment

What tiny environment tweak can you make today? Move biscuits out of sight, prepare fruit for afternoon snacks, keep a water bottle on your desk?

What to eat when life gets busy

When your schedule is full, convenience usually wins. But convenience doesn't have to mean unhealthy. The key is to rethink your definition of fast food: pre-boiled eggs, hummus with carrots, frozen vegetables, canned beans, or pre-cooked quinoa can all be turned into a healthy meal in minutes. By keeping simple staples on hand, you can build meals around what's quick, easy, and good for you.[9]

Decision fatigue is real. After making hundreds of decisions throughout your workday, choosing what to cook can feel like the final straw. This is where fallback options and preparation come in handy. Having a few easy go-to meals you enjoy can take the pressure off when decision fatigue is high and energy is low.

Smart cooking for busy schedules

- ✓ **Cook once, eat twice (at least)**: double recipes and portion into single or family servings; label with dish and date; freeze. Keep freezer grab-bags to avoid last-minute takeaways.
- ✓ **Set and forget shopping**: use a grocery delivery service with a recurring basket (eggs, yogurt, tinned beans, pre-cooked grains).
- ✓ **Create a list of your favourite 10-minute meals**: reduces decision fatigue on your busiest days.

Challenges of shift work nutrition habits

If you work shifts, whether in healthcare, hospitality, or transport, eating healthily becomes more complex. When your body clock is disrupted through work schedules or long-haul travel, mealtimes become inconsistent, and food options are limited, especially late at night. Food vending machines are not known for their delicious, nutritious, healthy eating options. Even if your schedule is irregular, your approach to fuelling can be consistent.

Shift-friendly nutrition hacks

- ✓ **Prepare grab-and-go meals**: prepare overnight oats, boiled eggs, wraps with hummus and veg, or protein-rich snack boxes that include nuts, seeds, and fruit.
- ✓ **Prioritize hydration**: keep a refillable water bottle nearby to sip regularly and limit caffeine in the latter half of your shift.
- ✓ **Front-load protein and slow carbohydrate**: eating protein-rich meals earlier in your shift can support sustained energy and help prevent sugar crashes.

What if you struggle with your weight?

Weight is influenced by many factors such as hormones, sleep, stress, and genetics. It's not just dependent on food choices. Here, the focus is on nourishment, energy, and habit-building, not restriction. The goal is not a number on the scale but sustainable wellbeing: stable energy, sharper focus, and more balanced mood. Healthy weight often follows when healthy habits are in place.

If you've struggled with food in the past, it's easy to carry guilt or shame around your choices. But habits change best in an environment of self-compassion, not criticism. Judgement doesn't create change, strategy and kindness do.

Reflection moment

When you think about your eating habits, are you encouraging or critical?

If a friend spoke to themselves the way you do, how would you respond to them?

Finding your nutrition fit at work

Workplace culture often revolves around lunchtime takeaways, birthday cake, or after-hours drinks. These moments can feel tricky to navigate when you're trying to eat in a way that supports your energy. But building healthy eating habits doesn't mean opting out of connection. It just means preparing to choose differently.

Start with small, intentional swaps: bring healthy options to share, decide on a one-drink limit, or have a nourishing meal before social events so you're not relying on what's on offer. These aren't restrictions, they're boundary-setting tools that protect your choices without isolating you.

Progress through consistency

The good news is that change doesn't require a dramatic overhaul. It starts with simple, intentional habits that fit into your day. Over time, these micro-habits build up to form sustainable change. Progress is about being prepared, staying consistent, and treating yourself with kindness.

As Nick's story shows, small changes in how you eat can dramatically shift how you feel. When you begin to experience more stable energy, sharper focus, and fewer mood dips, you begin to see that better nutrition isn't about giving things up; it's about the small habits you repeat consistently.

And if you're unsure what's really making the difference, that's where honest reflection and wearable data can help. Tracking subtle physiological shifts, like energy levels, HRV, or sleep quality, helps you see how your body responds to what, when, and how you eat. These patterns help you tune into what truly works and let go of what doesn't.

What your wearable tells you about Your Nutrition Habit

Most devices estimate total energy (calorie) expenditure, by adding an estimate of your resting energy (based on age, sex, height, and weight) to activity energy inferred from accelerometers and heart rate signals. The absolute numbers aren't perfect, but the patterns over time help you gauge output and make smarter fuelling choices.

Some wearables offer integrated food logging, while others sync with apps to allow AI-powered photo logging and even glucose monitoring to show how meals affect blood sugar and recovery.

The goal isn't to obsess over numbers but to use your wearable, whether it's nutrition balance, calories in/out, or meal-fuel effects, to guide simple adjustments that align with your wellbeing goals. Think of it as having a personalized feedback loop: *Are your meals supporting your focus in the afternoon? Is your hydration influencing your recovery overnight?*

To help you apply this practically, let's break down key wearable insights across three critical points in your day: morning, afternoon, and evening. You'll learn how small tweaks to food and hydration choices can make a noticeable difference in your performance, energy, and recovery.

Morning: What's your body saying before breakfast?

Your morning data can offer clues about how your body handled the previous day's nutrition and hydration and how ready it is to face the day ahead.

- **Elevated RHR**: if your RHR is higher than usual in the morning it may be a sign that your body is still working hard to recover. Possible triggers include dehydration, a heavy or late-night meal, caffeine or alcohol intake, or stress.
- **Daily readiness score**: consistently low readiness scores first thing in the morning can be a sign your system is under strain and not fully recovered. Triggers often include poor sleep quality, processed foods, or unstable blood sugar from the previous day.
- **Sleep quality and duration**: a full night's sleep paired with a low recovery score can be a red flag. Reflect on your choices from yesterday:
    - Evening meal: Was it too heavy, too late, or missing key nutrients to support rest (e.g. protein, fibre, magnesium-rich foods, think leafy greens, nuts, seeds, and wholegrains, all rich in magnesium to support better sleep)?
    - Caffeine timing: Did you have caffeine after 2 p.m.?
    - Hydration: Were you adequately hydrated? Did you drink alcohol (even one or two drinks can fragment sleep)?

Afternoon: What happens after lunch?

The afternoon is often where nutrition blind spots show up. Wearables can help you catch the early signs of blood sugar crashes, dehydration, or stress overload.

- **HRV dips**: a noticeable drop in HRV after lunch can signal strain, often linked to refined carbohydrates, processed foods, excessive caffeine, or dehydration.
- **Low daily readiness score**: not eating enough (common when skipping meals during busy days) can create an energy deficit. This can show up as reduced resilience and poor recovery.
- **Elevated RHR**: even mild dehydration reduces blood volume, which means your heart must work harder to circulate blood. This can show up as an elevated RHR compared to your baseline, especially if you're not ill or overly stressed.

Evening: How did the day add up?

Your evening wearable data reflects how well your body handled the day's demands and can be influenced by your nutrition choices.

- **HRV before bed**: if your HRV is lower than usual it may reflect cumulative strain from poor hydration, excessive caffeine, or low-level inflammation in response to stress or diet.
- **Sleep latency** (time to fall asleep): struggling to fall asleep can be linked to a late heavy meal, sugar spikes, alcohol, or too much caffeine in the afternoon.
- **Readiness score**: if your readiness or recovery score is lower than usual and your sleep, activity, and stress levels haven't changed, it could be your body signalling the need to prioritize rest and recovery.

Reflection moment

How often do you connect what you eat or drink with the way you feel? What patterns stand out in your wearable data, like RHR, sleep scores, or readiness scores?

Your nutrition breakthrough

Just as wearables help you spot patterns in your heart rate, recovery, or sleep, self-reflection helps you tune into how your body responds to the food you eat. If you don't use a wearable, a simple practice of noticing what, when, how you eat, combined with how it makes you feel, is an accessible way to build awareness. If you do use a wearable, this kind of reflection complements your data beautifully, helping you connect subjective experience with physiological feedback.

As you know by now, this isn't about calorie counting, weighing food, and keeping a detailed food diary. It's about tuning into your body with curiosity and learning to listen for the signals it's sending; your framework for this is the 'Aha Model'.

Awareness: Using a food diary to spot what's missing

You often assume you're eating 'well enough', but busy schedules, skipped meals, and mindless snacking often leave the body under-nourished, without even realizing it. When you're on the go at work, lunch gets sidelined, caffeine becomes a stand-in for meals, and snacks are consumed on autopilot between tasks. Over time, these habits create subtle nutritional deficits that erode energy and resilience. You might be getting enough sleep, but if your cells aren't being properly nourished, your energy won't be replenished.

Using the 'Aha Model' of habit change lets you build awareness of not only what you're eating but also how energized you feel.

Use the following questions to reflect on yesterday's nutrition and hydration:

- *Did you wake up energized or sluggish?*
- *Did your meals include protein and slow-releasing carbohydrates?*
- *Did you drink water regularly throughout the day?*
- *Did you notice any change in mood or clarity between lunch and late afternoon?*
- *Was your last meal light and balanced or heavy and rushed?*
- *Did you hydrate in the evening, or rely on alcohol to unwind?*

Reflection moment

What lessons have you learned through honestly reflecting on your eating habits?

Habit: Fuelling for better nutrition and energy

Now that you've built awareness of your current eating patterns, it's time to identify specific nutrition habits you can adopt to create meaningful change. The goal is simple: design habits that fit naturally into your day, not ones that feel like extra work. Each part of your day offers opportunities to steady energy, sharpen focus, and build resilience. Use the following strategies as a guide to select habits that match your unique requirements.

Morning: Set the tone for energy and focus

What you do first thing in the morning creates the foundation for how you think and feel throughout the day. Habits to consider:

- ✓ **Start with hydration**: drink a glass of water before your first tea or coffee to rehydrate and kick-start digestion.
- ✓ **Prioritize protein at breakfast**: add eggs, Greek yogurt, or a protein smoothie to reduce mid-morning energy dips.

✓ **Add fibre-rich carbohydrates**: include oats, berries, or wholegrain toast to sustain focus through the morning.

Afternoon: Maintain energy and mental clarity

Afternoons are often when energy slumps, cravings, and decision fatigue kick in. Be mindful of your second or third coffee; its impact can last well into the evening. A few well-timed nutrition strategies can help keep you steady. Here are three suggestions:

✓ **Eat slow-digesting carbohydrates at lunch**: choose lentils, wholegrains, or vegetables to support blood sugar balance and reduce the post-lunch crash.
✓ **Include a source of protein**: tofu, tuna, chicken, or eggs help support focus and stress resilience.
✓ **Plan an afternoon snack**: pack a protein-rich snack like hummus and carrots, roasted chickpeas, or a boiled egg to stay energized without relying on caffeine or sugar.

Evening: Support recovery and prepare for tomorrow

Evening nutrition isn't just about winding down; it's about setting your body up for overnight repair and next-day energy. Habits to consider:

✓ **Finish eating 3 hours before bed**: this gives your digestive system time to rest and reduces late-night cravings.
✓ **Taper fluids in the evening**: set a reminder to stay hydrated without overdoing it right before bed.
✓ **Choose a light, nourishing snack if needed**: try oatcakes with almond butter or a handful of walnuts if you feel peckish late at night. This helps stabilize blood sugar and supports restful sleep.

Action: Making nutrition habits stick

Once you've picked a habit, pause to check it's the right one for you. Choose something that resonates with you; choose a food you'll enjoy adding to your meal preparation and, of course, make the new habit simple and repeatable. That's where habit stacking comes in.

Habit stacking involves pairing a new habit with an existing one, allowing new habits to integrate seamlessly into your day. It was popularized by James Clear in *Atomic Habits* and it taps into your brain's natural desire to associate specific cues with set routines.[10] Instead of creating habits in isolation, habit stacking weaves them into what you already do, reducing mental effort and increasing the chances of long-term success. A simple formula for habit stacking is: 'after [current habit], I will [new habit]'.

Stack your habits

- ✓ **After** clicking the kettle on, **I will** prepare a healthy lunch.
- ✓ **After** each online meeting, **I will** take a large glug of water.
- ✓ **After** brushing my teeth, **I will** grab some healthy snacks for mid-morning.

Start with one nutrition habit. Anchor it to something you already do daily. By anchoring new habits to well-established ones, the brain associates them as part of the same sequence, reinforcing adherence and making habit formation feel effortless. The key is making your new habit part of an existing routine. And to help it stick, track your progress, not to judge, but to acknowledge and build confidence in your new routine.

When it comes to improving nutrition, many of us fall into the trap of trying to change everything at once. We overhaul our diet, ditch all our favourite foods, and aim for perfection from day one. But neuroscience tells us this approach rarely works. As journalist and behavioural science author Charles Duhigg notes, big changes often fail because they rely on motivation, a fleeting resource that's difficult to sustain.[11]

Small, consistent habits build real change

Instead, it's the small, consistent habits that create real, lasting transformation. Unlike motivation, which comes and goes, habits are automatic. They're ingrained in our daily routines, requiring less effort over time. This is why high performers, from elite athletes to successful entrepreneurs, rely on systems of habits rather than willpower alone.

When you ask your brain to juggle too many changes at once, you trigger resistance and your mind defaults to what's familiar, even when it doesn't serve your wellbeing. This is especially true with nutrition, where habits are often linked to comfort, culture, and emotion. Instead of aiming for a complete dietary overhaul, focus on one simple, specific habit and stack it onto an existing routine.

Like Nick, your breakthrough comes from small, consistent shifts, not dramatic rules. Use your wearable data or reflection check-ins to choose one habit to test this week. When you build habits around nourishment, not restriction, change sticks.

Reflection moment

What are you hoping to achieve from your new habit? How will you know your habit change has been successful?

Nourish to flourish

Your nutrition isn't just about fuelling your body; it's about fuelling your life. The food and drink choices you make each day shape far more than your physical health. They influence your energy, focus, emotional resilience, sleep quality, and ability to perform under pressure. A key takeaway from this chapter: your next meal is an opportunity to fuel not just your body, but also your focus, calm, and clarity. When approached intentionally, nutrition becomes one of your most powerful wellbeing tools.

What you've explored in this chapter isn't a list of restrictions, rules, or rigid plans. It's a mindset shift from fuelling to 'get through the day' to eating in a way that helps you show up at your best. The tools and strategies are designed to be simple, flexible, and sustainable. Change doesn't come from doing everything at once; it's about doing one thing well.

You've seen how steady changes like Nick's, can lead to powerful results. Whether it's swapping a pastry for a protein-rich breakfast, drinking water between coffees, or eating meals that balance energy instead of spiking it, the key is choosing habits that fuel rather than drain you.

With the right fuel, your body recovers more efficiently, your brain performs more effectively, and your stress response becomes more resilient. Nutrition is only one part of your wellbeing toolkit; sustaining performance also means creating space in your day to breathe, think, recover, and protect what matters most.

In the next chapter, you'll explore balance, what it really means, why it's essential for sustainable high performance, and how to find it amid the demands of daily life. You'll learn how to identify your stress triggers, create better boundaries, and build deliberate moments of recovery. Because wellbeing isn't about doing more, it's about making better choices with the time and energy you already have.

Stabilize your energy

- ✓ **Make smart swaps**: choose minimally processed options over sugary convenience snacks (e.g. nuts and berries instead of biscuits, a 10-minute stir-fry with frozen veg or pre-cooked grains instead of a takeaway).
- ✓ **Build balanced meals**: prioritize protein, fibre, and healthy fats at each meal to slow carbohydrate absorption and stabilize blood sugar. Think fish/chicken/eggs/Greek yogurt/tofu and vegetables, wholegrains and legumes.
- ✓ **Keep meals regular**: for most people, regular, balanced meals beat grazing. If you snack, make it protein and fibre-led (e.g. yogurt with seeds, hummus and vegetable sticks) rather than sugary or ultra-processed food.
- ✓ **Space them out**: many people do well with about 3–5 hours between meals to allow digestion and stable fuel release. Adjust for training load, medication, or pregnancy.
- ✓ **Minimize ultra-processed foods**: these are linked with higher calorie intake and increased risk of heart disease and Type 2 diabetes. Favour whole and minimally processed foods most of the time.

4

Your Balance Habit

Deadlines don't pause for school pickups. Stress doesn't clock off at 5 p.m. And personal responsibilities don't wait politely for your inbox to clear. Trying to give equal time to everything creates a brittle lifestyle, one that doesn't flex with real life. And when the scales tip, as they inevitably do, you don't just feel behind, you feel out of control.

This isn't just your story. It's the story of modern work and life. Across industries, professionals from ambitious entrepreneurs to senior leaders are navigating longer hours, blurred boundaries, and a culture that rewards constant availability. What was once a clear divide between professional and personal time has dissolved, replaced by a cycle of rushing, multitasking, and the pressure to always be *on*. The constant pace is taking its toll with rising stress, eroded energy, and burnout, even among high-performing, outwardly successful teams and individuals.

Why balance matters more than ever

It should come as no surprise that a global Deloitte study found that over 77% of professionals report feeling burned out in their current roles, with 91% saying stress negatively affects the quality of their work. The top causes of stress include unmanageable workload, lack of support, and the inability to switch off.[1] The impact of constant stress without recovery goes far beyond performance. It drains energy, disrupts focus, unsettles your mood, and undermines long-term health.

No wonder so many of my clients ask: *Why does it feel like there's never an off-switch, not at work, not at weekends, not even on holiday? Will I ever get back a sense of control?*

The answer is 'yes', but it requires a different approach. One that steps away from the outdated ideal of work–life balance and embraces something more flexible, realistic, and personal.

In this chapter, you'll explore how finding your unique work–life fit, rather than striving for perfect balance, is the key to reducing burnout risk, managing stress more effectively, and showing up at your best. You'll gain insights from high-performance sport and psychology, and through the story of Beth, a 42-year-old senior executive whose life looked balanced but felt exhausting in reality. You'll see how even small shifts can lead to meaningful change.

Meet Beth: Silently slipping toward burnout

On paper, Beth's life looks like a perfect example of work–life balance. A senior marketing executive in the pharmaceutical industry, she has the kind of career many would envy. She is respected by colleagues, leads major campaigns, and is steadily climbing the corporate ladder.

At home, she has two children under ten and a supportive partner with his own demanding job in tech. She makes time for family, shows up to school events, manages a consistent gym routine, and even tries to squeeze in a few mindfulness sessions using an app each week. Their household runs on routines, logistics, and a colour-coded family calendar with every detail mapped from morning drop-offs to Zoom calls and after-school activities. It's like a work of art with every hour accounted for.

No matter how much Beth accomplishes, she ends every day exhausted and slightly anxious, as if something has been forgotten or someone has been let down. Even downtime feels performative. While she makes time for family dinners and gym classes, these moments begin to feel like boxes to tick rather than genuine time for connection or restoration.

At work, she worries she isn't being strategic enough. Her internal dialogue is a constant stream of 'you should be doing more'. Her workdays bleed into her evenings, and her weekends are often hijacked by unfinished tasks. She's physically present but her thoughts are stuck in work mode, unable to switch off.

Her breaking point comes on what should be an ordinary Thursday morning. Her child's school calls unexpectedly; he's unwell and needs collecting. At the same time, she has a client presentation due in 90 minutes. She reschedules the presentation for the next day, cancels her afternoon calls, leaves work, picks up her son, skips lunch, and spends the day looking after him. Once he's finally asleep, she returns to her laptop and works into the night, finishing just after 1 a.m.

'I was trying to control everything so precisely, but it was breaking me,' she later told me. 'I had the title, the income, the family life. I'd built a life that looked balanced on paper, but I wasn't living it. I was managing it. I began to feel like I was failing at everything.'

That week, Beth books an appointment with her GP. The ongoing pattern of work pressures spilling into her personal life, low energy, poor sleep, and recurring minor illness is finally given a name: burnout. Her GP's first recommendation is simple but powerful: stop. Step away from the source of pressure. When we begin working together, the first step is allowing her system to recover. From there, she gradually begins to rebuild the routines and boundaries that support her wellbeing and resilience for the long term.

What she needs isn't a better schedule. It's a shift in how she defines success; one built around energy, not just responsibilities.

Beth isn't alone. Her story reflects a growing reality for many professionals: they're performing well but living poorly. Their calendar is full, but fulfilment is low. The balance may look good externally, but internally there's a growing disconnect, and no amount of colour-coded planning can fix that.

That's why we need a different approach; one that supports the fluid, messy, wonderful reality of modern life, and helps us move from striving for balance to designing fit. Beth knew this all too well. She was trying to manage a perfectly scheduled life, ticking every box, and still felt like she was dropping the ball. What she discovered, through burnout and recovery, is what many professionals are realizing: balance isn't about equal time; it's about protecting what matters most.

The myth of work–life balance

You've seen the image: a perfectly balanced scale with work on one side and personal life on the other. The idea is simple: give both equal time and you'll achieve balance. But in reality, this model sets you up for stress, guilt, and constant pressure to *fit it all in*.

Instead of feeling in control, many of my clients feel stuck, either sacrificing their personal life to stay on top of work or stepping back from their career goals in search of a balance that never quite arrives. Striving for this unattainable balance can lead to more emotional strain, especially for high-performing professionals who are already stretched.

What imbalance feels like

- ✓ **Overwhelmed**: a workload that consistently exceeds your available time or energy.
- ✓ **Exhausted**: exhaustion from constantly adjusting schedules to meet external demands.
- ✓ **Inadequate**: a growing sense that no matter how much you do, it's never enough.
- ✓ **Guilt**: feelings of guilt or failure for not maintaining 'perfect' routines.
- ✓ **Disconnected**: a loss of community, working in isolation or under constant pressure.

Finding work–life fit

The idea of **work–life balance** is not just unrealistic; it's outdated.[2] It assumes that work and life are two separate forces to be evenly managed. But for most modern professionals, that picture doesn't hold. Life is too dynamic, demanding, and interconnected for rigid ideas of balance.

Work–life fit isn't about equal time; it's about aligned energy. It's about creating a rhythm that works for you, not one that just looks good on paper. This flexible and integrated approach has been shown to support greater wellbeing, resilience, and job satisfaction across a wide range of roles and industries.[3] In the next section, you'll explore how to achieve work–life fit and how this simple shift can help you to reclaim your time, protect your energy, and feel like yourself again.

Reflection moment

Are you giving more than you have to your workplace, colleagues, network, and finding there's nothing left for you?

How would you know you gave too much?

Work–life fit is about finding a pattern that aligns with your available energy, current life circumstances, and values. In essence, it's about designing a life that fits you, not forcing yourself to fit into an outdated model of balance.[4] Work–life fit allows for flexibility when life gets messy, and adaptability as needs and priorities shift. Rather than striving for the elusive work–life balance, work–life fit invites you to ask: *What works for me, right now?*

The mindset shift

Psychologist Carol Dweck's pioneering work on mindset shows that our abilities aren't fixed, they can grow through effort, reflection, and support.[5] This includes not only how you learn, but also how you manage time, energy, and stress.

When you approach your life with a growth mindset, you stop chasing an unrealistic picture of balance and instead focus on making decisions that reflect your needs, energy, and life as it really is. Life doesn't have to look perfect to work well for you. What matters is creating a rhythm that flexes with your needs.

Career development experts Helen Tupper and Sarah Ellis highlight three mindset principles that can help you build this rhythm: accepting, knowing, and understanding.[6]

Accepting that life won't always be evenly balanced frees you from guilt when compromises need to be made. *Knowing* your non-negotiables keeps your focus on what matters most, so your energy isn't spread too thin. And *understanding* that fit is personal helps you avoid the comparison trap. What works for a colleague may not work for you, and that's okay. Once you recognize your energy patterns and responsibilities, you can let go of what you think you 'should do' and instead design a schedule that works for you.

Beth's identity had long been tied to high expectations in work, parenting, even in wellbeing habits. Letting go of perfection and embracing flexibility didn't come easily. But as she began to shift her inner dialogue from 'I should be doing this' to 'I'm learning how to live differently,' she unlocked a more compassionate, adaptive version of herself.

That shift didn't come overnight. There were tears, missteps, and days that still felt heavy. But there was also a new foundation forming. A quieter confidence. A sense of self-trust. She was no longer trying to get back to the old Beth. She was building something new, a version of herself with more space, and far less guilt. It's not a shortcut around struggle. It's the decision to move through life differently.

Learning to fall up

Life has a way of knocking us off course. For high achievers, the fall can feel especially disorienting, because so much effort has been poured into avoiding it. You plan, you anticipate, you prepare. And yet, at some point, something will tip the scales. A family crisis, conflict at work, a period of ill-health. But what if those moments weren't setbacks? What if they were springboards for building resilience?

Positive psychologist Shawn Achor calls this mindset shift '**falling up**': the idea that the most resilient people don't just recover from adversity, they turn it into a stepping stone.[7] During times of stress or crisis, most people instinctively search for a way back to how things were. But those who thrive find a different path: the path up.

When adversity is met with a growth mindset it can become a spark for growth, insight, and even transformation. This isn't about toxic positivity or pretending everything's fine. It's about learning to respond to difficulty in a way that stretches you, rather than shuts you down.

Beth's story reflects this in a deeply human way. She came to realize that taking the time to recover from burnout wasn't the end of her professional identity; it was a new path. Letting go of the need to be perfect gave her permission to be honest, with herself and with others. She opened up to her team. She worked with her husband to rethink how they shared the load at home. She redefined what work–life fit meant for her, not in terms of hours worked or plates spun, but in how connected, calm, and energized she felt at the end of the day. Positive psychology calls this reframing 'a cognitive pivot', and it's the foundation of falling up.

Reflection moment

How can you reframe a recent challenge as a turning point, not a failure?

Reframe challenge

People who are most resilient in the face of stress make a conscious mental pivot. They learn to see setbacks not as failures, but as signals for growth. When you start to view stress as a signal, not a threat, you give yourself the chance to respond with clarity rather than panic. That shift in thinking can make all the difference.

Beth began to practise this by viewing her burnout not as a character flaw, but as data. It wasn't a sign of weakness; it was feedback from her body and mind that something had to change. This shift from self-judgement to self-inquiry allowed her to pursue change with kindness, rather than criticism.

If you're going through a period of work that feels too full, too fast, or just too much, know this: there's nothing wrong with you. You haven't failed. You may be standing at the point where the old way of living is no longer sustainable. And that's a powerful place to begin again. It's often the time when people *should* reach out for help, but failure to notice the signs or read the data sends them dangerously close to burnout.

Next, you'll look at the science behind stress and recovery, and the evidence-based tools that work to reset your nervous system, boost resilience, and help you find calm amid the noise. You'll learn how to spot your early-warning signs and start to protect the essentials in your life: time, attention, and wellbeing.

Rethinking stress and burnout

From the moment you wake to the time you fall asleep, some form of stress will cross your path. Stress is inevitable but it's not always harmful. That may sound surprising, especially if you've faced relentless deadlines, emotional demands, or the weight of keeping too many plates spinning. Instead, it's not the stress itself that determines the outcome, it's your relationship with it. As Carol Dweck's growth mindset theory shows, stress can become a catalyst for growth rather than a drain on your resilience.[8]

Workloads increase, family responsibilities demand your attention, and unexpected events throw your routines off course. But while you can't always control what's coming, you can learn to work with it. By building a framework that protects your energy and supports recovery, you can navigate challenges without becoming overwhelmed.

The key is not avoiding stress but knowing how to move through it fully. That's where the stress cycle comes in and why it matters so much for your wellbeing.

Inside your stress response

The stress cycle is rooted in decades of research on the human stress response which is governed by two separate biological systems.[9] The first is the autonomic nervous system which acts as your body's rapid response team. It activates the sympathetic nervous system, your 'fight-or-flight' response, and your body moves into a state of high alert. Heart rate rises, muscles tense, breathing quickens, and blood flow is redirected to prepare you for action.

When stress persists, the second biological system that is activated is the **HPA (hypothalamic-pituitary-adrenal) axis**. Here your brain signals the release of cortisol that sharpens focus and mobilizes energy, helping you stay alert under pressure. While essential in short bursts, chronic activation of the HPA axis is a major biological pathway linking stress to burnout.

The stress response is useful in the short term as it helps you respond to a challenge, but it's meant to switch off once the challenge has passed. If you don't signal to your body that the threat has passed, the stress cycle stays open, draining energy and disrupting sleep, mood, and long-term health.

When stress doesn't switch off

This is one reason why you might finish your workday yet still feel wired, edgy, or mentally overloaded hours later. Your tasks may be done, but your body hasn't received the message that it's safe to stand down. You're left 'tired but wired'.

Completing the stress cycle isn't just about stopping the stressor; it's about sending clear signals to your body that it can return to safety. That signal might come through movement, deep breathing, laughter, human connection, or rest. These recovery cues are essential, yet they're often the first things to go when life gets busy. And when those cues are missing you don't recover, you accumulate stress. That's when stress becomes chronic, and burnout risk increases.

Reflection moment

Think back to a recent stressful day. *Did you give your body a signal that the challenge had passed, or did you carry the stress with you into the evening?*

Banish burnout

Burnout doesn't always start with a crisis. More often, it creeps in quietly, disguised as tiredness that doesn't go away, focus that flickers, and a creeping sense that no matter how hard you work, it's never quite enough.

Psychologists Christina Maslach and Michael Leiter describe burnout as a chronic mismatch between the individual and the resources available.[10] It's not about a lack of effort. In fact, it's often the opposite: burnout tends to strike those who care deeply and try hard, but who are working in a system that's out of sync with what they need to thrive. Many organizations are working to adopt more flexible ways of working, not to create perfect balance, but to help people find a better fit between their energy, values, and responsibilities.[11]

Nearly one in three employees globally report symptoms of burnout, and rates are especially high among younger professionals and career changers, who are often navigating steep learning curves, unclear boundaries, and the pressure to prove themselves.[12] That's why recognizing and responding to burnout early is a critical skill, not just a wellbeing issue, but a professional strength.

Burnout red flags: What to watch for

- ✓ **Physical signs**: persistent fatigue, frequent headaches, muscle tension, disrupted sleep, or frequent illness.
- ✓ **Emotional signs**: irritability, feeling flat or detached, loss of motivation, or a sense of dread about work.
- ✓ **Cognitive signs**: brain fog, difficulty concentrating, forgetfulness, slow decision-making.
- ✓ **Performance signs**: feeling less effective despite working harder, struggling to prioritize, losing satisfaction in achievements.

Healthy boundaries

Burnout is not a personal failure. It's a warning sign. A signal that something in the system must change, and the earlier you respond, the better the outcome, for your health, happiness, and long-term wellbeing.

This is where boundaries become an act of self-respect, not restriction. They help you reclaim energy that would otherwise be lost to fatigue, multitasking, and the mental clutter of trying to do everything at once. Healthy boundaries should not be viewed as indulgences; they are strategically preventing you from burning out.

Boundaries that help protect your balance

- ✓ **Time boundaries**: protect time in your calendar for deep work.
- ✓ **Task boundaries**: whenever possible say 'no' to non-essentials and give each task a clear start and finish.
- ✓ **People boundaries**: communicate availability, delegate responsibility, and set expectations early to avoid last-minute pressure.
- ✓ **Place boundaries**: create distinct zones for focus, collaboration, and rest.

The point of these strategies isn't to add more to your to-do list. It's to take some things off. Not all at once but with just enough intention that you start to feel the difference.

For early career professionals or those in a new role, this shift can be particularly challenging. Early in your career there's a strong pull to say 'yes' to everything, and to always be available. But real impact doesn't come from running on empty. It comes from creating a system that supports your energy, resilience, and wellbeing over time.

You're allowed to pause.

You're allowed to recover.

And when you do, you don't lose your edge, you sharpen it.

From burnout risk to recovery

As Beth reflected on her work–life fit, she realized she was caught in a cycle, giving more than she had, constantly trying to meet other people's expectations, and leaving little space to rest, recover, or recalibrate. She was over-performing on every front yet still felt like she was falling short. It wasn't just the hours. It was the mismatch between what was being asked of her and the resources she had to meet those demands.

Once her burnout was recognized and she finally had the space to step away from the pressure, the breakthrough came. Recovery began with an honest look at where her energy was being drained, and where she could begin to rebuild it.

Beth began doing something she'd never thought she had permission to do: she began saying 'no'. Each 'no' became an act of self-preservation, not from a place of resistance, but from a commitment to her wellbeing. She realized that saying 'no' wasn't about letting people down. It was about showing up more fully for the things that mattered most.

Reflection moment

Which activities or commitments matter most to you and how could you create consistent time for them?

What your wearable tells you about Your Balance Habit

It's easy to miss the early signs of imbalance until they become impossible to ignore: poor sleep, constant fatigue, short tempers, or that gnawing sense of being constantly *on*. But what if you didn't have to wait until burnout hit to make a change? What if you could see the warning signs earlier and respond with insight instead of letting pressure build?

That's the value of wearable technology. It confirms what you might not be consciously aware of; it's an early-warning sign of what your body already knows, and what you may have been trying to ignore. Let's take a closer look at the metrics that matter most for balance, what they tell you about stress, and how to interpret them if you're using a wearable.

Resting heart rate

Your resting heart rate (RHR) is an indicator of how your body is coping behind the scenes. It is highly responsive to both physical and emotional load. When it's consistently elevated, even slightly, it can be a signal that your system is under strain. An RHR increase of 5–10 bpm above your personal baseline, especially first thing in the morning, may indicate that your body is under-recovered or fighting off fatigue, illness, or hidden stress.

A low RHR isn't always a cause for concern, particularly in well-trained individuals. However, if your RHR drops to an unusually low level *and* you feel light-headed, fatigue or unwell it's worth speaking to a health professional.

What to look for:

- **Sustained elevation**: Is your RHR consistently elevated compared to your personal baseline (especially during sleep)? This may be a sign to rebalance workload, recovery, and stress.
- **Positive response**: Does your RHR return to baseline or decrease following periods of good sleep, hydration, rest days, or lower stress? If so, that's a sign your recovery strategy is working. Well done.
- **Temporary spikes**: Are you seeing short-term spikes in RHR after late nights, alcohol, illness, or stress? It's natural to experience occasional spikes, they're not necessarily a bad thing and are to be expected, especially if the body is responding to a temporary stressor. The key is whether your RHR returns to baseline over the next day or two.

Sleep duration and quality insights

When it comes to recovery, sleep is where your body does its deepest repair work. But good sleep doesn't just happen. It's shaped by your habits and, most importantly, your boundaries.

Most wearables provide a sleep score which typically combines factors such as total sleep time, time in each sleep stage, RHR, heart rate variability (HRV), and movement to estimate sleep quality and recovery. The higher the score, the better your body is at bouncing back. In the context of work–life fit, this matters. If your evenings are blurred with late-night emails or mental overload, your sleep score will show it, often before you consciously feel the effects.

What to look for:

- **Total sleep time**: Are you consistently getting at least seven hours per night? Less than that over time is linked to energy dips, irritability, weaker immune function, and reduced cognitive performance.
- **Deep sleep**: Are you spending enough time in the deeper stages of sleep? This stage is most strongly linked with physical restoration, tissue repair, and memory consolidation. Poor boundaries in the evening, like late screens or work stress, can reduce time in these stages.
- **Fragmentation**: Is your sleep fragmented by frequent wakeups or high movement? This could reflect stress, alcohol, late meals, or an overstimulating evening routine.

Heart rate variability

Of all the wearable metrics available, HRV is the gold standard for understanding how your body is coping, especially when it comes to long-term stress and burnout risk.

In short, HRV tells you how adaptable your nervous system is. In a healthy system, the two branches of your autonomic system, your sympathetic, 'fight-or-flight' response and your parasympathetic, 'rest and digest' mode, work like a well-balanced see-saw, responding to pressure when needed, then returning to a calm, restorative state. But when you're constantly under pressure, without enough recovery, the balance tips. You're stuck in the stress cycle. Over time, this can leave you feeling exhausted, anxious, or emotionally flat, classic symptoms of burnout.

What to look for:

- **Trend over time**: Is your average HRV staying stable, improving slightly, or trending downward over days or weeks? Trending downward is not a good sign.
- **Night-time recovery**: Is your HRV higher overnight, especially during deep sleep and on less stressful days? That's a sign of better health, flexibility, and resilience and shows that your body can recover efficiently when under pressure.
- **Fluctuations**: Are there noticeable drops in HRV after poor sleep, high workload, emotional stress, or travel? It's normal for HRV to fluctuate day-to-day. Downward trends over several days are a signal to step back, dial back intensity, and recharge.
- **Recovery habits**: Can you spot the habits that help raise your HRV, such as meditation, time outdoors, regular movement, or quality sleep? These patterns reveal what best supports your nervous system.

HRV is highly individual, and absolute values matter less than trends relative to your personal baseline. If your HRV stays low even when you're resting, it may be a sign that your nervous system is stuck in a stress response, unable to fully shift into recovery mode. This suggests that you're operating in a state of chronic strain, even if you're no longer aware of it.

This is why I pay particular attention to HRV when working with clients who *feel* fine but suspect something's off. HRV is often one of the first physiological indicators that chronic stress and burnout may be developing beneath the surface.

Daily readiness score

In the context of work–life fit, daily readiness score is a powerful tool. It gives you permission to adjust, not push through every day on autopilot. A lower score might be a signal to scale back where you can, protect focus time, or prioritize recovery strategies. A higher score? That's your green light to lean in and make progress on the things that matter most.

What to look for:

- **Guidance**: How can your daily readiness score guide your day? Use it to inform, not dictate. A low morning readiness score might mean moving a tough meeting to tomorrow, taking more mindful breaks, or choosing a walk instead of a high-intensity workout.
- **Patterns over time**: Are there clear patterns? Can you link lower readiness scores to disrupted sleep, excessive travel, or stress? Can you spot when better boundaries or habits help raise your score?
- **Feel vs data**: Does your score reflect how you *feel*? If you feel *fine* but your readiness is low, that may be a sign you're running on adrenaline, not true recovery.

Your readiness score reflects how your lifestyle is supporting your recovery. It doesn't replace intuition; it sharpens it. Over time, it helps you balance effort and recovery in a way that's not just reactive, but intentional.

Beth's wake-up call in numbers

For Beth, her data became both a wake-up call and a motivator. When she first began tracking her HRV, she noticed it remained consistently low, even after quiet weekends, sleeping seven hours, and what she thought was rest. Her body wasn't bouncing back. It was a wake-up call that what she was experiencing wasn't just tiredness, it was physiological depletion.

As she began protecting boundaries and building in new habits, her morning walks, a non-negotiable 7 p.m. cut-off from emails, her screen-free transitions, her HRV slowly improved. She noticed how her readiness scores tracked alongside HRV trends. That insight gave her something far more powerful than information. It gave her hope.

This kind of feedback is transformative. It takes wellbeing out of the realm of vague good intentions and into something concrete, measurable, and motivating. It's not about tracking for the sake of numbers. It's about using insight to make choices that support your energy, focus, and ultimately, your work–life fit. For Beth, it was the difference between giving up and keeping going.

If wearable devices help you measure stress objectively, reflective practices bring you back into your own experience. Together they create self-awareness that truly drives change.

Your balance breakthrough

Burnout rarely arrives without warning. The body whispers before it shouts. The trouble is, you're often too busy to hear it. That's why building in moments of reflection can be so powerful, not as another task, but to stay connected to how you're *really* doing. Through journalling you create your personal dashboard, a space where you can start to spot trends that may have been invisible before.

By now, you'll be familiar with the 'Aha Model', the framework you've used throughout this book to turn insight into meaningful, sustainable action. You've seen how awareness, habit, and action work together to make your habits stick, especially when life is busy. The goal isn't to do everything. It's to do *one thing* that makes everything else feel a little lighter.

Awareness: Identify your balance gaps

Building awareness of your work–life fit begins with noticing the habits, patterns, and pressures that are quietly draining your energy. These simple check-in prompts help you tune into your mood, track your energy, and identify where small, targeted shifts could make the biggest difference.

- *When do you feel most focused, calm, or energized during the day?*
- *What tasks or moments drain you, emotionally, physically, or mentally?*
- *What feels unsustainable in your current routine?*

When you tune in, you start protecting your day based on what your body needs. If you feel depleted, it's not failure, it's feedback. Your system is asking for adjustment. This is where compassion becomes action.

Non-negotiables: *Commitments that matter most*

- ✓ **Morning calm**: five minutes to breathe, journal, or move before checking your phone.
- ✓ **Hydration**: carrying a water bottle and committing to drinking throughout the day.
- ✓ **Movement**: a ten-minute walk at lunchtime or a stretch break between meetings.
- ✓ **Boundaries**: turning off work notifications after a set time.
- ✓ **Connection**: calling a friend during the commute home.
- ✓ **Rest**: finding time for pause after work, even for five minutes.
- ✓ **Sleep**: a consistent bedtime even if your evening schedule is unpredictable.

Habit: Embed balance in your routine

Choosing a personal non-negotiable isn't just about getting through a difficult week; it's a powerful act of self-compassion. It's a commitment to honouring your needs in a world that often pulls you in ten directions at once.

When you consistently protect one small habit, whether it's eating a proper breakfast, stepping outside for fresh air, or shutting your laptop by 6 p.m., you begin to rewire your internal dialogue. You stop saying, 'I'll rest when everything's done', and start saying, 'I matter. My energy matters. My future self matters'.

The key is choosing a non-negotiable that fits *you*; one that aligns with your needs, values, and current capacity. There's no single right answer, only what restores your clarity and sense of control.

> **Reflection moment**
>
> *If your future self could thank you for one action today, what would it be?*

Action: Create habits that stick

Action creates change, but for a habit to truly stick, it needs more than willpower. Psychologist Wendy Wood has shown that habits are not formed by intention alone, but by what you do repeatedly in a stable context.[13] The right cue, a behaviour that's easy, and an environment that supports it are the building blocks of habits. In other words, if you want your new wellbeing habit to last it should fit naturally into your day, and feel like part of your *real* life, not just your ideal one. The key isn't more effort, it's smarter design.

Wood's research also demonstrates the difference between goals and habits. Goals engage your conscious mind, but habits rely on **environmental cues** and **repetition**. Under stress, time pressure, or fatigue, motivation often collapses. But automatic behaviours, carried out almost without thinking when triggered by consistent cues, keep going. That's why one of the most effective behaviour change strategies is to anchor your new habit to something you already do.

The more you link your habit to something you already do, the easier it becomes to sustain without added effort. These cues become mental shortcuts, allowing the behaviour to happen without needing a fresh decision every time. This is the power of **sticky habits.**

Sticky habits

- ✓ **Move**: leave your walking shoes by the door and step out for five minutes when you finish work.
- ✓ **Sip**: as the kettle boils, fill your water bottle and take five sips.
- ✓ **Stretch**: after your morning meeting, take a two-minute gentle stretch at your desk.
- ✓ **Clear**: when you close your laptop, tidy your workspace for tomorrow.
- ✓ **Reflect**: keep your journal under your pillow and before sleeping write one line of reflection.

If you find consistency tricky (which is completely normal), you can gently layer in **accountability**, not as pressure, but as support. That might mean a weekly check-in with a friend, sharing your new habit with a colleague, or journalling how you feel after doing it. The key is to protect your progress without punishing yourself for imperfection.

Reflection moment

What's something you already do that could act as a natural cue for habit change?

Find your rhythm; reclaim your energy

The old model of work–life balance no longer matches the pace and pressure of modern life. Work–life fit invites you to design a life that adapts with you, not against you. It offers flexibility when life feels messy, and clarity when everything is pulling at your attention. It's not about splitting your time equally; it's about making conscious choices that reflect what matters most.

Balance isn't a destination. It's finding a rhythm that evolves as your life, values, and energy change.

Your ideal work–life fit won't look the same in every stage of life. In fact, it's meant to evolve. Some periods will be work-heavy, maybe you're leading a major project, changing career, or building a business. Other stages might require more space for parenting, caregiving, recovering from illness, or needing space to breathe, whatever you need.

Work–life fit embraces fluidity and encourages conscious choice, not constant guilt. For example, you might have a period that requires high work intensity and low personal demands. That may be the time to lean into growth and ambition. On the other hand, you might be managing health issues, family transitions, or burnout recovery. That's the time to prioritize restoration and simplicity wherever possible. There's no *perfect* place on this scale, just the place that's right for you *right now*.

Beth's story reminds us that over-scheduling and high performance doesn't always lead to fulfilment. For years, she tried to make her days look balanced, keeping every plate spinning, holding her diary together with colour-coded precision. But what she discovered was that she didn't need tighter scheduling, she needed stronger boundaries.

She began with a simple question: *What do I want to protect in my week*?

That led to a short list of non-negotiables, family dinners three nights a week, walking meetings on Wednesdays, and a clear 'digital sunset' each evening. None of these were radical changes, but they created space for recovery. That space gave her room to breathe, think clearly, and reconnect with her values. Her energy, mood, and leadership performance improved, and she began to feel more like herself again.

Your new work–life fit can start the same way, not with a dramatic overhaul, but with one deliberate change; make it a habit and then build on it. Maybe it's saying 'no' to a task that drains you. Maybe it's carving out five minutes of silence before your day begins. Whatever you choose, trust that it matters. Because when your energy is protected, your impact grows, not in spite of your wellbeing, but because of it.

Embrace a rhythm that restores you. And when that rhythm is supported by rest, not just downtime, but real replenishing recovery, something powerful happens. You stop chasing energy and start restoring it. That's the focus of the next chapter, where you explore how quality rest and recovery fuels not only wellbeing, but performance, capacity, and long-term resilience.

Keep balance flexible

- ✓ **Don't get too rigid**: if you have a rule to 'never check email after 6 p.m.' treat it as a principle you flex when life gets messy. Avoid guilt by adjusting as the week unfolds.
- ✓ **Spot early-warning signs**: notice persistent fatigue, irritability, or difficulty sleeping, then course-correct (lighter evenings, buffers between meetings, a short to-do list).
- ✓ **Name what's outside your control**: list what you can't influence, then shift focus to what you can (boundaries, asking for support, clearer priorities).

5

Your Rest Habit

Rest isn't just recovery; it's how your brain stays sharp. Your brain performs best in rhythmic cycles of effort and renewal. Without regular pauses, synapses fatigue, attention narrows, emotional regulation falters, and creativity dries up. Short, intentional breaks restore the systems that drive focus and problem-solving by down-shifting the body from a stress-biased state into a calmer, more resourceful one. Think of it as sharpening the signal and quieting the noise in your mind.

Modern work crowds out these cycles. Long hours, packed calendars, and a full inbox have become the hallmarks of success. Constant context-switching, notification noise, and meeting overload create a drip-feed of stress that feels normal, until it isn't. Burnout isn't too much work; it's the result of *how* work is designed today. While total hours may have remained steady, intensity has surged through digital overload, tighter deadlines, and constant demands on attention.[1] Recent workplace trends show employees face up to 275 interruptions a day across email, chat, and meetings, creating an infinite workday.[2] This constant cognitive load leaves little room for focus or creativity and makes the idea of having time to rest feel like a distant dream.

The answer is to design your effort so that recovery is built in. Rest is not time away from performance; it's part of performance. When you plan it, you optimize cognition, protect your energy, and make your highest-value work easier to sustain.

The power of the pause

If you've ever called IT support for a faulty device, you'll know the first question they ask: '*Have you tried turning it off and on again?*' Your body works in much the same way. You aren't designed for constant uptime. Just like your smartphone needs to recharge, your nervous system, brain, and emotional reserves need regular resets to run well.

You wouldn't expect your phone to last three days without charging, or to run optimally with every app open at once. Yet that's exactly how many professionals treat their bodies and minds: always *on*, rarely recharging. They push through warning signs, override the need to pause, and wonder why they feel flat, foggy, or unmotivated.

And beneath this surface-level productivity lies a deeper truth. You're not burning out because you lack capacity, you're burning out because your capacity is stretched in the wrong ways. A growing body of evidence shows that burnout is less about total workload and more about insufficient recovery.[3] The result is an exhausted workforce that is constantly active but increasingly ineffective.

In this chapter you'll discover why rest is not the opposite of work; it's the foundation that makes great work sustainable. Drawing on neuroscience, physiology, and psychology, you'll explore how intentional rest can unlock the focus, creativity, and resilience needed to thrive in today's demanding world. You'll also meet Rachel, a passionate business owner who learns first hand that building rest into her day doesn't slow her down; it gives her the capacity to keep leading with energy.

Meet Rachel: From always *on* to intentionally rested

Rachel, 52, runs a thriving physiotherapy practice, known not just for its clinical excellence, but for the warmth and care she brings to every interaction. Her patients adore her. Her team trust her. She is the anchor, the one everyone counts on. Driven, generous, and deeply committed, Rachel wears many hats: business owner, mentor, clinician, mother, daughter, friend. And she wears them all well.

But something doesn't feel right. Her days blur into evenings. Her phone is rarely out of reach. Even during holidays, she's checking messages, fielding questions, filling in the gaps. Every Christmas, without fail, she comes down with flu-like symptoms. 'It's like my body collapses the moment I stop,' she says. 'I spend my holidays recovering, not enjoying them.'

Rachel starts to feel increasingly hollowed out. Her mind races through the night. Her energy dips unpredictably. Even when she takes time off, she struggles to rest. She's not burned out, but she can see the cliff edge; what she doesn't appreciate is how close she is to it.

What complicates matters further is that her workload isn't restricted to the office. Rachel has two teenage children, a supportive partner, and ageing parents who live nearby. She isn't their carer, but she is their emotional anchor. Her mum has started repeating stories. Her dad, once sociable and chatty, now seems withdrawn. 'I'm not sure what's happening, but I know I need to keep an eye on them,' she shares during coaching. 'I'm carrying this weight of responsibility all the time; it's exhausting.'

She's not just juggling deadlines. She's juggling care, concern, and constant mental load. What she fears most isn't failing, it's keeping this pace going and slowly losing herself in the process.

When we begin working together, stepping back feels like failure. But slowly, Rachel gives herself permission to pause. With support, she starts rebuilding her day with rest at the centre. She experiments with moments of micro-rest: a quiet start to the day, consciously pausing between treating patients, and a screen-free buffer before bed. At first, she resists; rest doesn't come naturally.

The feedback from her wearable changes everything. Once Rachel begins tracking her strain and recovery the numbers tell a story she can't ignore. That objective feedback becomes the catalyst she needs to start making small but deliberate changes. Within a month, her stress scores begin to shift. She can clearly see which recovery strategies work best for her. Even more significantly, her thinking clears, her energy stabilizes, and for the first time in a long while she begins to feel like herself again.

Rachel doesn't change everything. She changes what matters.

In this chapter, you'll learn the science and simple practices that helped Rachel stop viewing rest as something to earn and start treating it as something to build in. Rest gave her back her lightness, clarity, and calm, not by stopping, but by creating a rhythm that sustained her. It became her quiet superpower, the thing that made everything else work better.

Rest reframed

Rest fuels performance; it doesn't sit in opposition to work. It's the scaffolding that supports it, a fundamental biological and psychological requirement. Rather than viewing rest as the absence of productivity, it's time to understand rest as the driver for high-quality focus, emotional regulation, creativity, and sustainable output.

As you explored in the 'Your Movement Habit' chapter, the General Adaptation Syndrome (GAS) shows that stress is the signal and recovery is the upgrade. Deadlines, challenging work, and training all create a load. Recovery windows found in sleep, active rest, or lighter days, enable **supercompensation**, the period when your system returns not just to baseline but slightly above it. Skip the recovery and you stall adaptation; stretch stress for too long and you drift toward fatigue and diminished performance. In practice, schedule recovery to fit the workload.

The busy trap

Your difficulty with rest isn't just practical; it's cultural and psychological. Many of us have internalized the idea that stopping equals slacking. Stillness can feel uncomfortable. It disrupts the rhythm of visible productivity you've been taught to value. You may feel guilty, unproductive, or exposed. As Claudia Hammond notes in *The Art of Rest*, gentle, low-demand activities, like a short walk or bath, feel restorative precisely because they're small, doable acts of off-duty attention.[4]

Your brain needs periods of recovery to function optimally. Without rest, you default to reactive thinking. The prefrontal cortex, the brain's control centre for decision-making and focus, begins to falter. You shift from thoughtful to reactive. Mental fatigue clouds your judgement and intensifies emotional responses. Constant doing creates constant depletion.

Rachel experienced this first hand. On her first day of prioritizing rest she notices more anxiety, not less: 'It feels like I'm letting my team down.' But as she sticks with it, she notices a shift. Stillness brings insight. Her nervous system calms. For the first time in years, she feels clear-headed and grounded.

Reflection moment

What if your next breakthrough came not from pushing harder, but from pausing more?

What stops you from taking rest seriously and how might your productivity and wellbeing improve if you did?

The illusion of productivity

Activity isn't the same as progress. The optics of speed and constant availability can feel productive, yet the brain pays a hidden tax every time you switch tasks. Even brief interruptions can leave **attention residue**, a mental trace that clouds decision quality.[5] Fewer, deeper blocks of work almost always beat a day of fragmented tasks.

Strategic rest enhances focus, sharpens memory, stabilizes emotion, and increases adaptability, all vital skills in a high-performance environment. The science supports what elite performers have always known: without rest, focus deteriorates, creativity fades, and reactivity takes over.

In the workplace, however, this mindset is still catching up. Rest is often mistaken for laziness, or worse, weakness. Neuroscience tells a different story. Real rest is strategic. When harnessed deliberately, it can sharpen your thinking, reduce stress, and protect long-term capacity.

Your two-breath reset

A rapid way to downshift your nervous system is the **physiological sigh**. Popularized by Stanford neuroscientist Andrew Huberman, it is one of the most researched rapid-reset techniques. It's a natural breathing pattern your body already uses during sleep to restore calm.[6] Use it any time you feel tense, rushed, or overstimulated.

1. Inhale deeply through the nose.
2. Take a second, smaller top-up inhale to fully expand the lungs.
3. Exhale slowly and completely through the mouth, making the exhale longer than the inhale.
4. Repeat two or three times.

Tip: If you feel light-headed, pause and breathe normally.

The cost of always being *on*

Attention residue isn't the only cost of switching. Each time you jump tasks, your brain also treats it as if something is wrong. Cognitive neuroscientist Amishi Jha, known for her work on attention and task-switching, has shown that frequent task-switching activates the brain's error detection system. Even trivial shifts, like checking email mid-task or flicking between tabs, trigger a subtle stress response, signalling the brain that something is 'off'.[7]

You weren't designed to be constantly switched on. Endless emails, pings, tabs, and multitasking keep your brain in a state of low-grade hypervigilance. This sustained load doesn't just tire you out, it actively undermines your ability to think clearly. Working memory shrinks, problem-solving stalls, and emotionally you're more reactive and less resilient.

Over time, these frequent 'micro-alarms' chip away at your mental bandwidth. Clients often see this in their wearable data; activities they once considered mindless, like email checking or toggling between tasks, show up as measurable strain on their body's energy reserves. What looks like productivity is often neurological overload.

Rest, leadership, and capacity

Leadership means modelling recovery as much as managing tasks. Effective leaders know that cognitive clarity, emotional regulation, and strategic thinking don't come from being constantly switched on. They come from having the capacity to respond, not just the urgency to react.

Showing your team that pausing is a strength, not a weakness, sets the tone for enduring success. When leaders protect their own recovery, they send a powerful message: wellbeing and performance are partners, not competitors. It's not simply time off that restores you; it's the quality of rest deliberately built into your day.

Reflection moment

What would change if rest was part of how you measured performance, not just in yourself, but in those you lead?

Addicted to stimulation, but starving for rest

British physician and bestselling author Rangan Chatterjee highlights the tension many modern professionals face between constant stimulation and the absence of meaningful recovery. In *The Stress Solution*, he shows how our always-on digital habits and multitasking overload the nervous system, leaving us craving the next stimulation while starving for restoration.[8]

Chatterjee advocates for tech-free pauses, single-tasking, and creating simple daily rhythms that restore calm and reset the body. Like elite athletes who balance exertion with recovery, he argues that professionals perform best when they work in intentional cycles of effort and ease.

When your brain is flooded with stimuli, it doesn't get smarter, it gets noisier. Quiet the noise and you'll think more clearly, create with ease, and finish the day with energy to spare.

Deep work and strategic idleness

Daily recovery calms the nervous system, allowing the brain space to integrate and innovate. This is where computer science professor and productivity expert Cal Newport adds a behavioural and cognitive lens to the conversation.[9]

Newport shows how mental fragmentation, caused by constant emails, context-switching, and digital distraction, undermines your ability to think deeply, create meaningfully, and perform at your best. He argues that high performance isn't about doing more but about doing the right kind of work: focused, high-value tasks supported by intentional periods of rest.

Newport calls this **strategic idleness**: purposeful downtime that allows the brain to process, integrate, and innovate. It's in these quiet spaces, he suggests, that your most important insights emerge.

Lessons from high-performance sport

Just like muscles adapt through cycles of strain and recovery, capacity grows when you intentionally pair effort with restoration. The goal isn't to eliminate stress entirely (that's neither realistic nor helpful), but to build the awareness and habits that let you recover from stressful situations quickly, protect what matters, and stay grounded when life gets busy.

High-performance athletes understand this better than anyone. They face constant pressure to perform optimally, yet they don't push at full intensity every day. Instead, they structure their entire routines around **intentional strain**, followed by deliberate recovery to build their capacity.

They practise discomfort in measured doses, build confidence under pressure, and know that pushing too hard without recovery doesn't make you stronger; it wears you down.

You can learn from this. Treating every day like a sprint risks burnout. Treating your week like a training cycle creates the conditions for both focus and recovery. Plan clear peaks of effort and follow them with deliberate restoration through sleep, light movement, proper fuelling, reflection, and time in nature. Manage your load, prioritize recovery, and trust that consistent, purposeful rest is how capacity is built and protected.

Reflection moment

If you treat your week like a training cycle, where will you place deliberate peaks of effort and where will you find time for recovery?

Rest that restores

One of the most powerful effects of rest is its ability to shift your nervous system into a state of recovery. When you're constantly in motion, responding, reacting, pushing through, your body stays stuck in high alert. This stress state, governed by the sympathetic nervous system, is designed for short bursts of activity, not sustained strain.

Rest activates the parasympathetic nervous system, responsible for calming the body after periods of stress. This 'rest and digest' mode balances the high-alert, 'fight-or-flight' state that many professionals operate in for most of the day.

When you pause with intention, through practices like deep breathing, slow movement, or mindfulness, you help your body shift from a high-alert state to this restorative mode. This change slows the heart rate, reduces cortisol levels, and supports immune recovery. This isn't just about feeling better in the moment; it's about building your capacity to respond, recover, and perform. In the pages ahead, you'll find practical ways to weave rest into your daily routine, so rest becomes part of how you work, not just something you wait for. Once you understand which type of rest you're missing, you can begin building habits that fit with your day, not against it.

Choose the rest you need

These seven forms of rest, drawn from Saundra Dalton-Smith's book *Sacred Rest*,[10] highlight the many ways you can pause to recharge energy, reconnect with meaning, and restore a sense of calm.

1. **Physical rest**: your body needs both *passive* rest (sleep, intentional stillness) and *active* rest (light stretching, walking). Even a five-minute gentle yoga break can reduce tension and boost clarity.
2. **Mental rest**: when your mind feels overloaded, short pauses help quiet racing thoughts. Try two-minute scroll-free pauses, short breathing exercises, or quiet reflection between meetings.
3. **Sensory rest**: screens, noise, and notifications overstimulate the nervous system. Turning off alerts, using soft lighting, or closing your eyes for 60 seconds after screen time can reduce overload and support deeper evening recovery.
4. **Emotional rest**: naming your emotion reduces its intensity, 'name it to tame it'.[11] Taking even 30 seconds to acknowledge 'I feel anxious' or 'I feel frustrated' can help you shift gears and protect emotional energy.

5. **Creative rest**: when your thinking feels flat, step outside, listen to music, or notice something beautiful. Creative rest restores inspiration, especially when problem-solving or innovating.
6. **Social rest**: not all social interactions are energizing. For some, solitude is energizing; for others, connection is key. The important thing is knowing what recharges *you*.
7. **Spiritual rest**: this is about meaning. Through reflection, time in nature, journalling, or prayer, spiritual rest reconnects you with what truly matters.

Mindfulness: Stillness with a purpose

Mindfulness is the practice of paying full attention to the present moment, without judgement and without the need to fix or change anything. Far from being 'woo' or a fleeting wellness trend, mindfulness is a practical, evidence-based skill. Regular practice, even in short doses, has been shown to strengthen the prefrontal cortex, the brain's control centre, making it easier to focus, respond thoughtfully, and recover from stress.[12]

One of the simplest micro-practices is the one-minute body scan. It's quick, effective, and when used consistently, this mindful pause becomes a powerful habit for self-regulation and rest.

One-minute body scan

1. **Pause and breathe**: take a slow, intentional breath in through your nose and out through your mouth. Let your attention settle.
2. **Scan your body from head to toe**: gently bring your focus to the top of your head and slowly move down through your face, neck, shoulders, chest, arms, abdomen, legs, and feet.

3. **Notice**: without judgement, observe any areas of tension, warmth, fatigue, lightness, or discomfort. Ask yourself: *What's happening physically? What's happening emotionally?*
4. **Release**: if you detect tension, soften that area with your next exhale.

The pause that powers you

Non-sleep deep rest (NSDR) refers to practices that bring the body into a deeply relaxed yet awake state, supporting recovery without requiring sleep. In this state, the prefrontal cortex has a chance to reset. And because it can be done sitting down, it's easy to incorporate even in a busy day. Whether it's guided breathwork between meetings or ten minutes of visualization, they transform ordinary pauses into powerful anchors for recovery.

Everyday NSDR habits

- ✓ **Progressive muscle relaxation**: systematically tensing and then releasing each muscle group to release physical tension.
- ✓ **Guided breathwork**: using structured breathing patterns, such as box breathing or the physiological sigh introduced earlier in this chapter, to calm the nervous system.
- ✓ **Visualization practices**: mentally rehearsing peaceful scenes or positive outcomes to shift mood and focus.

Hot and cold: Sauna and sea as smart add-ons

I live on the Atlantic coast and while cold water dips aren't for everyone (me included!), a morning walk along the beach confirms that many people find it appealing. If these practices interest you, outdoor swimming, sea dipping, plunge pools, and similarly sauna can sit as optional add-ons to your wellbeing toolkit. Used alongside the recovery habits you've already found in this chapter, they can feel energizing, community-building, and often mood-lifting.[13]

Hot and cold exposures act as deliberate, controlled stressors that can help the two main gears of your autonomic nervous system shift more efficiently.

During exposure, both hot and cold typically increase sympathetic drive ('fight or flight'): you may notice faster breathing, a spike in alertness and a quickened pulse, especially in the first 20–60 seconds of cold. As you re-warm after cold or cool down after heat, many people experience a shift towards relaxation: looser muscles, steadier mood, and a pleasant post-session calm. In other words, the exposure is stimulating, and the after-phase is often settling. Responses vary by person, temperature, duration, and timing; treat this as an experiment, as outcomes vary.

Heat and cold: How to start

- ✓ **Cold (sea/shower/plunge pool)**: brief, safe exposure of 1–5 minutes, 2–4 times per week followed by a full warm-up. Keep it short at first and increase only if you feel well. Never go alone in open water.
- ✓ **Heat (sauna)**: short, comfortable sessions of 10–20 minutes, 1–3 times per week. Hydrate before and after. Exit early if light-headed.
- ✓ **Time it well**: schedule sessions at times when they won't disrupt sleep (morning swim, short stroll, and early light exposure are strong habit-stacking partners).
- ✓ **Begin gently**: start with lower intensity, shorter duration, less frequent exposures, allowing your body and nervous system to adapt safely.
- ✓ **Medical check**: if you are pregnant or have a medical condition, speak with a clinician first.

These habits can support daily recovery, but real restoration depends on a broader structure: nourishing food, movement you enjoy, and moments that downshift your system across the day. Whether you choose to add these to your wellbeing routine is up to you; there are plenty of ways to build a protective buffer that safeguards energy and creates space to recalibrate. In the next section, you'll learn how to put that buffer in place.

Protect the edges of your day

Creating intentional space at the start and end of your day is a strategic way to protect your attention, energy, and emotional wellbeing. Much like a moat around a castle, this boundary isn't about isolation; it's about defence. It protects your focus from being hijacked by urgency, distraction, or the weight of other people's demands.

As you've seen in earlier chapters, most people begin their day in a reactive state, checking messages before they've even got out of bed, diving into emails before breakfast, and blurring the line between work and rest. Over time, this lack of psychological transition leads to chronic cognitive overload, higher anxiety, and depleted resilience. A moat gives your nervous system space to shift gears, allowing you to enter and exit the workday with intention, not inertia.

Reflection moment

Where could you build in a moat in your day, not to do more, but to recover more effectively?

Boundaries that build recovery

Building a moat is a simple yet powerful habit, an act of self-leadership. You don't need hours of free time to feel more in control. Whether you work from home or commute, you need intentional boundaries at the edges of your working day.

Your morning moat might be ten minutes of guided breathwork (remember you need to get that morning light into your eyes, so step outside and take some long, slow, deep breaths), you could take up journalling, or take time to stretch before opening your inbox. Your evening moat might be a walk, a screen-free wind-down, or a short body scan to signal the close of your workday.

For many of my clients, their daily commute becomes a built-in moat, a natural transition space that offers a valuable opportunity to pause, decompress, and restore before stepping into the next part of the day. Whether in the car or on public transport, this in-between time can be reframed as a buffer zone between roles. Rather than filling it with emails or to-do lists, they reclaim it with small restorative rituals: listening to calming music, reading for pleasure, or calling a friend for a light-hearted chat.

Whatever form it takes, your moat is a commitment to your wellbeing and performance. It sends a powerful message to you and those around you that your energy is worth protecting.

Build a moat

Building a moat is one thing, protecting it is another. Without consistent boundaries, even the most well-intentioned rituals can be eroded by urgency, digital distractions, or competing priorities. Here's how to protect the space you've carved out for yourself:

- ✓ **Create a morning activation ritual**: before you open your laptop or join your first meeting, give your mind a moment to arrive. Try a tech-free coffee, a short walk, or uplifting audio. If you commute, use this time as a mental warm-up, something that energizes rather than agitates.

- ✓ **Build a shutdown ritual**: signal to your brain that the workday is complete. Review your to-do list, set intentions for tomorrow, and close your laptop with purpose.
- ✓ **Establish sensory cues**: the body and brain respond well to cues. Dim the lights, change into comfortable clothes, or light a candle to signal the start or end of your day. These rituals create a physiological and emotional shift.
- ✓ **Set tech boundaries**: the compulsion to check emails late at night or scroll first thing in the morning often comes from a place of anxiety. Start with gentle limits: move your phone out of the bedroom, delay your first check until after your morning pause, or create email-free zones (e.g. no inbox checks after 7 p.m.).

Media diets for mental clarity

Research by former CBS news anchor and positive psychology expert Michelle Gielan shows that watching even a few minutes of negative news can prime the brain for stress and reduce optimism for the rest of the day.[14]

With this in mind, Rachel reimagined her commute. Instead of driving to work listening to political news or phoning ahead to the practice, habits that used to heighten her stress, she began listening to uplifting music or audiobooks. These activities helped her arrive at work more energized and centred.

Her journey home followed the same principle: she used the evening commute to create a clear buffer between work and home life, whether it was silence, or a light-hearted podcast. These bookended pauses didn't just change her mood; they protected her capacity. 'I realized I was arriving home already overstimulated,' she shared. 'Now I use my commute as a space to de-compress before walking through the door.'

Whether you travel to an office or work from your kitchen table, every day offers a natural buffer between roles. How you use that moment matters.

Establishing **rest rituals** such as building a moat is a powerful start, but how do you know if they're really working? This is where wearable technology becomes a valuable ally helping you move from guesswork to objective data, showing whether your body is truly recovering and whether the rest habits you're building are having the impact you need.

What your wearable tells you about Your Rest Habit

Stress is often invisible, until it isn't. You might not realize how much strain your system is under until the signs are loud: disrupted sleep, brain fog, mood swings, low energy. For many midlife professionals, especially women, these symptoms can also overlap with the early stages of perimenopause, making it harder to know what's really going on.[15]

Just like your body sends cues through tension, fatigue, or irritability, wearables provide physiological feedback that can help you spot the signs earlier. When viewed through the lens of recovery, these tools show when your body is thriving and when hidden stress is beginning to take a toll. They turn invisible strain into visible signals.

For Rachel, this data was a form of validation. It confirmed the benefits of her new rest habits, her commuter moat, pausing between clients, screen-free evenings. Just as importantly, it flagged when old patterns started to creep back, allowing her to course-correct before slipping too far off track.

Let's explore the metrics that indicate your rest strategies are paying off. You'll find deeper guidance on sleep data, in 'What your wearable tells you about sleep' in the 'Your Sleep Habit' chapter.

Daily readiness score

Your readiness score acts like a daily check-in with your recovery system. Think of it as your daily compass, helping you make smarter decisions about how you work, lead, and show up. It gives you a clear answer to the question: *Is today a good day to push or to prioritize recovery?*

What to look for:

- **Morning scores**: if you have low morning readiness scores you may not be going into the day fully charged. Plan lighter cognitive work, slower mornings, or add extra rest practices in the days ahead.
- **Low scores despite good sleep**: if your readiness scores stay low even following a good night's sleep, it could be reflecting high strain from previous activity, stress, or emotional load.
- **Consistently low scores**: if you have low readiness for two or more days in a row you might be skimming the surface of rest without really recovering. Consistently low scores across several days can signal that your system needs a reset physically or emotionally.

Heart rate variability

For Rachel, low heart rate variability (HRV) revealed a hidden pattern: even when she was technically resting, if she hadn't mentally or emotionally unwound, her body stayed stuck in 'fight-or-flight' mode. The numbers reflected what she couldn't always articulate.

Once she began building her moat, switching off in the evening and limiting evening emails, her HRV began to rise. These upward shifts, though subtle, validated what her body had been trying to tell her all along: rest was working.

What to look for:

- **Drops in HRV**: a drop in HRV may indicate accumulated strain, poor sleep, or insufficient recovery, even if you feel 'fine'.
- **Stress-related changes**: pay attention to drops in HRV after high-stress days or poor sleep and use these signals as prompts to lean into your recovery practices.
- **Persistent lows**: if HRV remains low despite rest, it may point to deeper stressors such as emotional load or unresolved sleep quality issues.

Real-time heart rate

While resting heart rate gives you a big-picture view of recovery over time, your real-time heart rate, the number you can see live on your wearable, is a powerful tool for tracking how your body is responding to rest in the moment.

Whether you're taking a mindfulness break, finishing a stressful call, or walking after lunch, your live heart rate shows whether you're coming down from stress, staying activated, or slipping into calm. Tuning into this real-time biofeedback strengthens the link between what you *do* and how you *feel*.

What to look for:

- **Before and after checks**: compare your real-time heart rate before and after a mindfulness session, slow mindful walk, or rest strategy. A noticeable drop suggests your nervous system is shifting from *on* to *rest*.
- **Micro-pauses**: even when you don't feel different, short pauses may register physiologically. Your heart rate may show signs of recovery before your mind notices it.
- **Lingering elevation**: a high heart rate that lingers after a meeting or commute may signal the need for a longer buffer, perhaps a few extra minutes of stillness or deep breathing.

What's clear from the clients I've worked with, and the data I've analysed, is that your metrics mean little without knowing the story behind them. Even without a device, you can gauge how well you're resting by paying attention to what recharges you and what drains you.

Your rest breakthrough

Your energy levels, sleep quality, mood, and ability to focus are powerful daily indicators of how well your body is recharging. A reflective journal can help you connect the dots between how you feel and what your body is showing you. This is where insight becomes wisdom, and where rest becomes truly personal.

Let's use the 'Aha Model' to show how you can begin recharging your battery in a way that's realistic, restorative, and grounded in everyday life.

Awareness: Where is your energy leaking?

Awareness isn't about judgement; it's about understanding your need for rest more clearly. Without it, you stay stuck in the cycle of overwork and under-recovery. With it, you create the space to rest differently. The first step is tuning into *where* your energy is being drained and *what* your body is trying to tell you.

You've tracked how rested you feel, now ask yourself: *Where are you pushing through when you should be pausing?* Gaining the rest advantage isn't about doing more, it's about doing less, better. Build awareness through the following morning prompts to create an energy forecast for your day and use the evening journal prompts to build pattern awareness and plan rest for tomorrow.

Morning prompt:

- *How charged do you feel this morning: 100%, 75%, or running on low?*
- *What's one thing you can do today to protect or restore your energy?*

- *What signals is your body giving you right now: tension, calm, heaviness, fatigue?*
- *What pace feels right today: fast and focused, or slow and steady?*
- *How will you create a small moat today, a five- or ten-minute pause just for you?*

End-of-day prompt:

- *Did you take a real pause today, or did you move from task to task?*
- *When did you feel most clear, calm, or restored? What helped you feel that way?*
- *What drained you more than expected, and how might you recover?*
- *How would you describe your internal battery: charged, flat, or somewhere in between?*
- *What's one rest ritual you want to try tomorrow and what will you let go of?*

Habit: Choose one small act of recovery

Once you've noticed where your rest is missing, the next step is to create a habit that restores you. This isn't about overhauling your life. It's about choosing one practice that gives you the greatest return on recovery and committing to it consistently.

Sustainable rest doesn't only come from long holidays or spa days; it's built through small, consistent pauses that you protect, just for you. These scheduled non-negotiable moments might involve a five-minute pause between calls, a short stroll after meetings, or a screen-free wind-down before bed.

Reflection moment

What do you need right now to feel restored and to show up as the version of yourself you want to be?

Action: Rest that reflects who you're becoming

Now that you've pinpointed the rest habit that matters most to you, it's time to turn intention into action.

James Clear reminds us that habits are the compound interest of self-improvement.[16] Just as small financial investments grow steadily over time, small daily habits, repeated consistently, lead to meaningful, measurable growth.

This principle mirrors what high-performance sport has long understood. Under the leadership of Sir David Brailsford, British Cycling rose to world dominance by applying the theory of **marginal gains**: the belief that if you improve every area of performance by just 1%, the cumulative impact can be extraordinary.[17] From sleep and nutrition to tyre pressure and team communication, what mattered was optimized.

In the same way, rest builds through small, repeatable actions. One small moment of rest, repeated consistently, can reshape not just your levels of stress but your energy overall. If you want to feel calm under pressure, less stressed, and more emotionally present, the habits that get you there don't need to be dramatic, they just need to be repeated.

Reflection moment

When was the last time you gave your brain a real break, not a scroll, not a distraction, but space to reset? How did it feel and what happened to your clarity or mood afterwards?

Redefine success through rest

Let's be honest: in fast-paced workplaces, rest can still feel like a luxury. But what the science shows, and what stories like Rachel's confirm, is that short, intentional pauses are the most effective way to access the parasympathetic state, your body's built-in recovery system. Just five to ten minutes of breathwork, a mindful walk, or unplugged silence can restore the clarity your work deserves.

Too many professionals wait until they're exhausted, overwhelmed, or completely depleted before they finally rest. But as this chapter has shown, rest isn't a reward, it's a resource. One that fuels focus, sharpens creativity, regulates emotions, and sustains performance.

Working with high-performing professionals, one of the most common challenges isn't time, it's permission. You know you need to rest but feel guilty taking it. The moat gives you a structured way to claim that space without apology.

Rest is not about slowing down for the sake of it. It's about recharging to meet the demands of your day with clarity and strength. It's about pausing not because you're falling behind, but because you value what comes next.

Rachel didn't reclaim her energy through one bold change. She built it gradually, through consistent rituals at the edges of her day. Her morning commute became an anchor. An evening stroll became her permission slip to pause. Over time, these small habits reshaped her resilience.

If you've ever felt like your day runs you, rather than the other way around, this is your chance to shift that pattern. Start by building your moat and then protect it fiercely.

This isn't about being perfect. It's about being intentional. Every time you pause, you're not just resting, you're rebalancing, recharging, and reclaiming your capacity to perform with purpose. The real shift happens when you stop waiting for breaks and begin building rest into your life.

Protect your rest

- ✓ **Micro-mindfulness break**: pause for a one-minute body scan. Breathe deeply, scan your body slowly from head to toe, and release tension consciously. This activates your parasympathetic nervous system, reducing stress and enhancing cognitive function.
- ✓ **Screen-free meal**: enjoy your meals without screens. This aids digestion, reduces stress, and resets attention for the hours ahead.
- ✓ **NSDR break** (non-sleep deep rest): set aside ten minutes for guided relaxation. This technique restores dopamine levels, improves mood stability, and sharpens attention.
- ✓ **Sensory pause**: every hour, close your eyes or rest them from screens for one minute. Minimizing sensory overload protects concentration, reduces fatigue, and sustains cognitive performance.
- ✓ **Protect your moat**: guard the edges of your day. These crucial pauses prevent burnout before it starts.
- ✓ **Wind-down ritual**: spend 5–10 minutes journalling, organizing tomorrow's priorities, or tidying your workspace. This signals to your brain that the workday is done and supports psychological detachment.

6

Your Connection Habit

Connection happens in many forms: catching the eye of a trusted colleague during a tense meeting, a chance encounter with an old friend, a smile from a stranger, or a cuppa with a loved one. In those moments you feel seen, heard, and understood. It's a great feeling, isn't it? Yet it's something we tend to take for granted. With technology, connection is available at the touch of a button, 'I'll call them later', 'I'll check in via my socials'. It's never been easier to stay connected, yet many of us feel more alone than ever.

Whether you're introverted or extroverted, this chapter is for you. Connection doesn't mean constant peopling or noisy rooms; it means the right dose of the right relationships. Often smaller circles, deeper conversations, and intentional touchpoints protect your energy while strengthening your support.

This paradox of being surrounded, yet disconnected, is felt acutely in today's workplace. You might be part of a buzzing team, attending meetings, and curating a lively online presence, yet still feel a sense of disconnection from the very people you interact with. You're surrounded by notifications, not conversations. Busy with tasks but starved of relationships. And in the moments when support matters most, after a stressful day, over a quiet weekend, or when pressure spikes, you may find yourself asking: *Where are my people?*

This isn't a personal flaw or a failure to 'network better'. It's a systemic shift in how society and work are organized. Remote and hybrid setups, relocations for career opportunities, shifting relationships, and the demands of high-performance roles have redefined what connection looks like, and how easy it can be to lose. Many professionals, especially those early in their careers or living far from support systems, are navigating a landscape where professional visibility is high, but emotional support can be low.

Alone together: The new face of loneliness

Loneliness has become a silent epidemic of modern work. Former US Surgeon General Vivek Murthy highlights how **chronic social disconnection** increases stress, disrupts sleep, elevates cardiovascular strain, drives inflammation, and undermines workplace performance.[1]

The impacts show up in how teams relate and support one another: more absenteeism, presenteeism, and less engagement. Remote and hybrid environments are particularly affected as casual chats, coffee breaks, and shared laughter are replaced by online meetings and task-focused conversations. Digital tools may boost productivity but erode the spontaneous human moments that sustain belonging.

When meaningful connection is missing, your body doesn't just feel unsettled, stress response systems can stay more activated. Loneliness and isolation are associated with higher daytime cortisol and sympathetic arousal, making it harder for the nervous system to down-regulate. Sleep quality and continuity often suffer which can blunt the restorative processes linked to deeper sleep stages. Over time, this chronic strain increases vulnerability to fatigue, illness, and burnout.

Connection isn't optional; it's a core biological need. Loneliness is linked to a higher risk of premature death with effects spanning the cardiovascular, immune, and neurological systems.[2] Researchers often summarize this risk by noting that chronic loneliness can be as harmful to health as smoking 15 cigarettes a day.[3] This is why connection is a core component of sustainable wellbeing. Strong social bonds lift every area of performance, supporting emotional regulation, stress resilience, cognitive flexibility, and creativity.

Conversely, disconnection impairs decision-making, elevates stress hormones, and lowers productivity.

This chapter is your invitation to rethink connection, not as something passive or left to chance, but as a habit you can build. Through neuroscience, behavioural psychology, and real-world experience, you'll see how meaningful relationships fuel energy and resilience. You'll learn how to turn connection into one of your most valuable assets, especially if you're introverted, starting a new project, or returning from leave.

Meet Carina: Thriving in a new role but feeling disconnected

Carina is a rising communications specialist, working for a global brand known for its high-profile product launches. She recently landed her dream role in a vibrant new city, far from family and the university friends who know her best. The job is fast-paced and exciting, she's leading campaigns that make headlines, collaborating with smart, creative people, and earning real recognition for her work.

Carina identifies as an introvert. She enjoys being around people, but she recharges through calm, focused work and meaningful one-to-one conversations. In her hybrid role most interactions are task-focused but emotionally thin. Her days are full but not fulfilling. She rents a small studio on her own; the quiet helps after launch weeks but most evenings feel still rather than restorative. Weekends stretch longer without her old support circle nearby. By Sunday night, a sense of loneliness starts to creep in, reminding her she's building a new life at a distance from home.

Before the move, Carina had a close circle of university friends nearby, people she could call for spontaneous chats, venting walks, or celebratory wine-and-pizza nights. Now they're spread across cities and time zones their connection feels different. They still check in but the casual closeness of everyday connection has gradually faded, replaced by an emotional distance she hadn't anticipated.

It's not that her new colleagues aren't supportive. They're friendly, professional, and talented. But most conversations stay on the surface. It's collaboration without real connection and, over time, that leaves her feeling flat.

Carina comes to see me just before her 30th birthday. Milestone birthdays often trigger reflection and a reassessment of what's working, what's missing, and what needs to change. Like many people navigating life transitions, she isn't in crisis, but she knows something isn't right and she wants support to explore it. She feels exhausted in a way she can't explain. As we unpack what's happening beneath the surface, it becomes clear that one of the missing pieces is connection.

Her wellbeing hasn't unravelled overnight. It's the slow accumulation of emotional isolation in a time of transition, a pattern I often see in young professionals navigating new roles, new cities, and new identities. Carina feels like she no longer recognizes herself. And that's where we begin: by stripping back the layers to see what's truly draining her system.

She doesn't need a new job. What she needs is intentional, nourishing connection; the kind that recharges the **social battery**, not just ticks a professional box. She realizes that while she's working with a team, it's still collaboration without connection. And connection, she's learning, doesn't just happen, it has to be built.

Things begin to shift when she invites a colleague she feels comfortable with for a coffee. A moment of laughter and ease reminds her of who she was before loneliness crept in. They turn it into a habit, a weekly ritual. For someone with an introverted personality, this isn't just a pleasant break; it's a form of recovery.

Gradually, Carina's energy lifts. The work doesn't change, but she changes because she feels less alone in it. She stops questioning whether she's okay as she understands more about herself and her body's signals. Wearable data confirms the shift: deeper sleep, improved readiness scores, and steadier recovery patterns. The background hum of self-doubt: *Am I really happy? Is this sustainable?* fades. Her anxiety eases. She begins to trust her own signals again.

In the next section, you'll explore why connection isn't just a feel-good emotion or a company value. It's a vital ingredient for resilience and performance. You'll discover practical ways to build meaningful connection, even when time, energy, or confidence are in short supply. Because in the end, it's not about how many people you know, it's about how seen, supported, and connected you truly feel.

The science behind connection

You're used to being told to prioritize your physical and mental wellbeing, but there's a third pillar that underpins both: social wellbeing. At the heart of social wellbeing is connection, a multi-layered ecosystem ranging from family bonds to the restorative power of nature. Connection it turns out, isn't a single thing, it's multi-dimensional.

Evolutionary psychologist Robin Dunbar is best known for the concept of '**Dunbar's Number**', the idea that humans can comfortably maintain around 150 social relationships, structured in concentric circles: approximately five intimate ties, 15 good friends, 50 meaningful contacts, and progressively wider layers beyond that.[4] Each layer is needed to maintain psychological and physiological health.

Make your connection circles work

- ✓ **Audit for meaning**: if your days are filled with meetings but lack meaning, aim to add one human moment per day (a shared laugh, asking for help, check in with a friend).
- ✓ **Micro-touches count**: a short voice note or text can strengthen ties without draining time.
- ✓ **Protect your bandwidth**: kindly pause ties that consistently deplete and prioritize relationships that refuel you.

Wellbeing and performance outcomes are shaped not by how many people you know, but from the *quality* and *diversity* of your relationships. Building on this, Murthy outlines three essential dimensions of connection that contribute to our wellbeing.[5] These include an inner circle of trusted people who provide emotional safety and deep support; a second circle of social and professional colleagues, mentors, and peers who contribute to your sense of progress and shared purpose; and a third layer of acquaintances or 'weak ties', the barista who remembers your name, the neighbour you wave to, or a colleague who shares a laugh in passing. Each layer matters, offering distinct yet essential forms of connection. Though often overlooked, they play a measurable role in lifting mood, reducing loneliness, and reinforcing belonging.

Connection boosts your health

Connection also plays a vital biological role in your ability to manage stress, sustain energy, and even prevent disease. One of the most compelling pieces of evidence comes from the Harvard Study of Adult Development, an 85-year-long research project that continues today.[6] It found that the single greatest predictor of lifelong health and happiness isn't wealth, intelligence, or achievement, it's the *quality* of our relationships.

Participants who reported strong, supportive bonds lived longer, got sick less often, and experienced greater emotional resilience. By contrast, loneliness, especially the absence of one or two close, securely attached relationships, was linked to chronic stress, inflammation, and decline across cardiovascular, immune, and neurological systems. What jumps out from the findings is the stabilizing role of supportive relationships; emotional anchors you can count on when life gets messy or uncertain. In short, if you want to thrive and cope with the inevitable stresses of work and life, connection is essential.

The vital ingredient: Vitamin S

As you can see, meaningful relationships are not just psychologically nourishing; they're biologically protective. In fact, social connection is so fundamental to health that Dutch psychologist Paul van Lange calls it 'Vitamin S', a critical daily dose for the mind and body.[7] Just as vitamin C strengthens immune function, regular social interaction boosts resilience, buffers stress, and promotes healthier behaviours.

Wired to connect

Advances in neuroscience show we are hardwired for connection. At the heart of this are **mirror neurons**, specialized cells in our brain that help us interpret others' emotions and mirror them, enabling empathy and emotional synchrony. This is why our mood can lift after chatting with a positive colleague or sink when stress spreads through a team.

If you've ever shared an office with someone who drains the energy from the room, you'll know just how quickly one person's mood can ripple through a group. Whether you present yourself as calm and curious, or stressed and volatile, the impact has a contagious effect on those around you. The emotions you project, ripple outward.

These signals are amplified by **oxytocin**, often called the 'bonding hormone', which is released during positive social interactions. Even small gestures like eye contact, a warm smile, or a shared laugh, trigger oxytocin release. This not only boosts trust and connection but also reduces stress and strengthens feelings of safety and belonging.[8] So go ahead, share that funny anecdote, you might just be boosting your colleague's wellbeing as well as your own.

Reflection moment

What emotional tone are you projecting to those around you: calm, curious, supportive, or distracted?

The ratio that builds resilience

Even brief moments of connection matter. Psychologist Marcial Losada observed that high-performing teams tend to show more positive than negative interactions; summaries report higher averages (5.6:1) in top teams and below 1:1 in low-performing teams.[9] Treat this as a guide not a rule. **Constructive feedback** delivered with warmth, plus everyday positive exchanges, build resilience, trust, and team engagement. In contrast, persistent negativity erodes trust and stifles performance.

This insight is echoed in the research of psychologist John Gottman, who found that successful, long-lasting couples generally maintain a 5:1 ratio of positive to negative exchanges.[10] In other words, for every criticism or tense moment, five small acts of appreciation, interest, or empathy helped maintain trust and emotional balance.

The lesson extends beyond personal life. Whether in marriages or meetings, when negative exchanges outweigh positive ones, trust breaks down. The emotional tone you create through micro-interactions shapes how others feel and function. If you want your team to thrive, aim to highlight positives three to five times more often.

For Carina, making time for positive moments, sharing funny stories, and scheduling a regular coffee catch-up became more than a social gesture. Her energy shifted, her motivation was boosted, and she was reminded that connection isn't just comforting, it enhances performance for everyone.

Connection in a changing workplace

Hybrid and remote work have opened the door to flexibility, but they've also reshaped how and where you connect. For some, remote work offers a sense of focus and autonomy. For others, it can fuel disconnection or loneliness. What often gets overlooked is that your work environment doesn't just affect how you communicate; it directly shapes your social energy, the mental and emotional bandwidth you have available to build relationships.

In shared office settings, connection tends to be more visible and spontaneous. A corridor catch-up, a nod across the meeting table, or informal mentoring may seem small but these micro-moments matter. They build trust faster, soften stress, and remind you that you're not working alone. Team culture flourishes more easily when shared space reinforces psychological safety.

But there are hidden costs. Office environments can drain energy through constant interruptions, overstimulation, or the unspoken pressure to always be *on*. For some, especially introverts or neurodivergent individuals, these spaces may also prompt masking or emotional performance which can make everyday interactions more effortful and stressful.

Remote work flips the equation. It preserves focus and offers more control over your physical and emotional environment, which can feel protective during demanding periods. But it comes with its own stressors: a sense of isolation, fatigue from endless video calls, and the challenge of reading tone or mood through a screen.

Intentional connection in hybrid teams

Connection, not location, is the strongest predictor of engagement.[11] This calls for a mindset shift: connection isn't a side effect of proximity, but something that can be built intentionally. Whether that means carving out time for deep work followed by social check-ins, creating opt-in social spaces instead of 'forced fun', or checking in more informally, workplaces that prioritize connection are the ones where people thrive, not just perform.

Hybrid work is now the norm for more than half of professionals in the US and Europe.[12] One of the most effective ways to support connection in this environment is to design your working week around the strengths of each space. Use in-office days to nurture human connection. These are ideal for collaborative workshops, mentoring, or shared rituals that build team culture. Reserve remote days for deep, focused work, quieter reflection, or one-on-one check-ins that allow for more personal connection without distraction.

Rituals also matter, regardless of location. Whether it's opening meetings with a short check-in, celebrating small wins together, or using digital spaces for light-hearted interaction, these intentional touchpoints create a sense of rhythm and belonging. The goal isn't more meetings, but more meaningful ones.

When people feel genuinely connected, through shared space, mutual purpose, or psychological safety, they unlock resilience, motivation, and engagement. Belonging acts as both a buffer against stress and a bridge to stronger performance. In hybrid settings, where casual connection is less likely to happen by accident, building belonging must be intentional.

Reflection moment

Does your current work setup give you the right balance of focus and connection?

Who are the people, or what are the spaces, that help you feel seen, accepted, and supported?

The ripple effect of everyday interactions

This connection superpower is at the heart of what is known as '**The Ritz-Carlton Effect**', a principle described by Shawn Achor in

Before Happiness.[13] In the hospitality sector, outcomes depend on connection: staff are trained to lead with warmth, kindness, and attentiveness. One practice is the simple 10/5 rule: make eye contact and smile within 10 feet, then offer a friendly hello within 5 feet. These tiny habits spread through the environment and measurably lift experience when adopted in other settings.

Achor extended his research when he applied these principles to hospital settings. The results were striking: faster recovery rates, fewer readmissions, and higher staff satisfaction. When connection becomes part of culture, it enhances trust, lowers stress, and strengthens capacity to thrive. Imagine what a difference this could make to your organization.

Whether it's a five-star hotel or a hospital ward, the science holds true: people heal, perform, and connect better when surrounded by positive social cues. A warm smile, a remembered name, or a moment of empathy; these aren't extras; they're evidence-based, high-impact behaviours that shape how people feel, function, and flourish.

Creating positivity for performance

With a foundation of connection, a company creates a culture of **psychological safety**, enabling colleagues to feel safe in speaking up, taking risks, and being themselves. It's a vital condition for high performance; without it, even the best team-building initiatives fall flat. Psychological safety isn't built through grand gestures. It's built in everyday moments: how you open meetings, how you respond to feedback, how you make space for quieter voices.

By being the first to speak in meetings, you take the lead and set the social script from the first minute. Positive psychologist Michellle Gielan calls this the '**power lead**' because it shapes the emotional tone of an interaction from the start.[14] Opening a conversation or meeting with a brief, genuine positive cue, such as asking, '*what's one win you've had recently, big or small?*' sets a positive trajectory others naturally follow. These cues create social permission for optimism, collaboration, and engagement, creating a ripple effect through a team's culture.

Reflection moment

Think back to your last meeting or conversation. *How did you open it and what micro-shift would you try next time? (e.g. name a team win, ask an open question, or respond with solution-oriented language, 'let's build on that', 'what would make this easier?')*

Connection by design

Wellbeing isn't only shaped by how you spend your time; it's also shaped by *who* you share it with. Some relationships uplift you, spark energy, and leave you feeling more alive. Others, even when polite or necessary, can drain you.

The impact of relationships isn't the same for everyone. It depends on how you process the world, what restores or depletes your energy, and how sensitive you are to social dynamics. This is where the idea of a **social battery** comes in: the personal store of energy you bring to interactions. For some, connection is deeply recharging; for others, too much interaction can feel exhausting. Understanding how your battery works and how to protect and restore it, helps you build connections that sustain rather than deplete you.

Your social battery explained

We all have different thresholds for social interaction, and recognizing these differences is essential to protecting wellbeing. In the workplace, the wrong kind of interactions or simply too much interaction can erode your energy. Personality type will impact this: *Are you an extrovert or an introvert? Maybe a combination of both, an ambivert?*

Extroverts tend to feel energized by engaging with others. They often thrive in fast-paced, people-rich environments where collaboration and interaction are central to their day. They tend to enjoy large group settings and spontaneous social activities. Their outgoing personalities make them adept at initiating conversations; they find it easier to take the power lead in meetings. Let's hope the extroverts at your work have a positive mindset.

Introverts usually recharge through quiet time, reflection, or one-on-one conversations. Large meetings, group calls, or constant interruption can leave them mentally and physically drained. They often prefer smaller, more intimate settings where meaningful conversations can take place.

Neither style is better or worse, they're different lenses through which we experience the world. The key is to become more aware of what drains and restores you, then design your schedule accordingly.

Reflection moment

Are your daily interactions lifting you up, or wearing you down? What boundaries would help protect your social battery?

Finding the right connection

For Carina it wasn't just workload that drained her energy; it was the nature of her interactions that left her depleted. As someone who values depth and downtime, her social battery ran low in environments filled with surface-level chat or unstructured group time. Extended time in the open-plan office, plus meetings with mismatched communication styles, left her disconnected and fatigued. She described it as an **energy vacuum**.

In contrast, she felt lighter and more focused on days where she balanced solo work with time spent with people who energized her. Her breakthrough came when she shifted the question from, *How much connection do I have?* to, *What kind of connection restores my energy?*

That question helped her become more intentional about her social commitments. She began using a simple decision filter, if catching up with someone isn't a 'hell yeah' then it's an easy 'no'.[15] This simple decision-making process is about being honest with yourself; recognizing where your time and energy are best invested. By doing so, you begin to release the obligations and relationships that drain you.

Protect your social energy

Your Connection Habit is about tuning into your body's signals and designing your workday with care. Carina learned that even short bursts of overstimulation required longer recovery periods, and she's not alone. **Overstimulation** impairs executive function, increases anxiety, and reduces engagement over time. Ignoring these signs creates a social energy debt that's harder to repay.

Your ability to recover depends on many factors: personality, sensory thresholds, emotional load, even hormonal cycles.[16] Some days you'll bounce back quickly, on other days, even small talk might feel daunting. The key isn't to push through; it's recognizing your limits and responding with care.

Recognizing social overload

- ✓ **Mental fog after meetings**: you struggle to re-orient, re-read emails, or lose your train of thought.
- ✓ **Irritability and low patience**: you feel snappy or drained by mid-afternoon.
- ✓ **Body tension**: tight jaw/shoulders, headache, or shallow breathing during/after calls.
- ✓ **Withdrawal behaviours**: avoiding invitations, cancelling plans last minute, or multitasking through conversations.

Nature's pathway to connection

Connection isn't only built with people. It can also be restored in stillness, solitude, and the natural world. We're biologically wired to connect with the natural world, both the spaces we inhabit and the creatures we share them with. Whether it's a walk in nature or time spent with a pet, these connections calm the nervous system, regulate breath and heart rate, and shift us from stress into restoration. Nature offers space to breathe, think, and reset in an otherwise hyperconnected world.[17] It's also why that morning breath of fresh air you explored when building your morning routine is so beneficial for your wellbeing.

Safe spaces and emotional anchors

These restorative effects are strongest in places where you feel safest, especially at home and in your relationship with pets. Rangan Chatterjee speaks about the importance of 'safe spaces': environments that allow you to reset your nervous system and reconnect with what matters most. In his book *Happy Mind, Happy Life*, he highlights how the places where you feel most at ease are not just emotionally comforting, they're biologically restorative.[18] When you feel grounded and secure, stress hormones fall, heart rate slows, and your body begins to recover from the emotional load of daily life.

Home, when it offers this kind of safety, is more than a physical place; it's a protective buffer for the mind and body. That's exactly what Carina rediscovered. Returning to the family home at weekends offered something she hadn't realized she was craving: a sense of true belonging. Home was where the pace slowed, the sky felt bigger, and the pressure to perform lifted. She didn't need to explain herself; she could just be.

And waiting at the door, always, was Benji, her loyal dog, tail wagging as if she'd been gone for years. In those quiet moments, sitting beside him with no words, no expectations, something shifted. Her breath slowed. Her heart rate settled. She felt grounded again. In a world of noise and notifications, Benji reminded her what it felt to be deeply connected: no performance required.

The healing power of pets

Pet interaction can reduce stress hormones, increase oxytocin, and improve heart rate variability (HRV).[19] Whether it's walking a dog, stroking a cat, or even watching fish swim, pets offer connection without expectation. And you don't need a rural retreat or a golden retriever to experience this. Small nature-based rituals can nourish your system: watering plants, stepping outside between tasks, pausing by a window.

These moments in nature can be the perfect tonic when your social battery feels depleted. Balancing human and natural connection provides the reset you need to recharge at the end of a demanding day.

Reflection moment

Where do you feel most calm and connected: outdoors, with animals, or in moments of stillness?

What one small habit could you build this week that reconnects you with the natural world?

In earlier chapters you explored how daily habits leave a measurable physiological imprint; the same is true for connection. Wearable technology can reveal how social wellbeing (or the lack of it) shows up in your body through shifts in HRV, sleep quality, and recovery signals. The technology also offers innovative solutions for social sharing, accountability, and support. Let's take a closer look.

What your wearable tells you about Your Connection Habit

Wearable technology reflects the invisible cost of your social choices. Behind every heartbeat, every recovery phase, and every night's sleep lies a reflection of your emotional ecosystem. And connection, or lack of it, shows up in the data. By learning what your data says about your connection habits, you gain the power to shape them.

Real-time heart rate

Social disconnection, loneliness, or even subtle relational tension can activate the sympathetic nervous system, keeping your heart rate higher than it needs to be. You may not *feel* outwardly stressed, but your heart often tells a deeper story.

By contrast, emotionally safe, positive connection helps to activate the parasympathetic nervous system, promoting calm, regulation, and recovery. Even short moments of genuine connection can trigger this shift. It's the difference between doom-scrolling in the evening and sharing a meaningful call with someone who lifts you up.

What to look for:

- ♥ **Elevated heart rate**: Is your heart rate elevated during times that should be restful or low stress? Look for patterns, especially during evenings or after long blocks of solo work or social disconnection.
- ♥ **Calming connections**: Do you notice a calming effect after meaningful connection? Track your heart rate before and after check-ins, phone calls, or light, positive social interactions. A decrease may reflect emotional regulation and parasympathetic activation.

Sleep duration and quality insights

Your sleep is strongly influenced by your social connections. Many clients find that time with friends is uplifting and energizing, but that buzz can make it harder to wind down into restful sleep. Add alcohol to the mix and the disruption intensifies, further interfering with sleep quality.

It's a reminder that while connection is vital for wellbeing, it's important to be mindful of how certain activities can influence the quality of your recovery. Above all else, your wearable reflects how emotionally safe you feel. When your nervous system is calm, it's easier to slip into deep, restorative sleep.

What to look for:

- **Contrasting scores**: Do you have contrasting sleep scores between high-energy evenings out and relaxed catch-ups with a close friend? Compare your deep sleep duration or overall sleep scores after varying social occasions.
- **Emotional load**: Take note of your sleep quality and duration after social events: conflict, masking, or forced connection can impair sleep as much as physical exertion.
- **Night waking**: Do you wake more often after tense or demanding social situations? Elevated stress hormones may be disrupting overall sleep recovery.

Daily readiness score

Your body gives you cues every day about how ready you are to engage, focus, or connect. On your wearable this shows up as a daily readiness score based on a combination of resting heart rate, HRV, movement, and sleep.

When you feel socially nourished, safe, and supported, your body shifts into a calmer, more resilient mode. Your 'battery' is charged. When connection is strained or missing, stress signals linger longer and readiness drops. Even if you don't consciously notice, your device will.

What to look for:

- **Unexplained dips**: Do your scores fall despite good sleep and no major exertion? Consider whether emotional strain or social disconnection may be keeping your system in low-grade stress mode.

- ♥ **Boosts from support**: Do your readiness scores improve after time with people who make you feel safe, supported, or understood? Notice the connection between meaningful moments and your body's recovery.
- ♥ **Impact of rituals**: After a calm conversation, time in nature, or gentle social rituals, do you notice your readiness scores rise? That's your nervous system signalling restoration.

Technological features that boost social connection

Wearable and wellbeing platforms offer features that go beyond personal tracking. Tools like activity sharing, group challenges, and progress updates enable you to stay linked with family, friends, or colleagues. Sharing progress fosters accountability, builds community, and creates support systems that help you stay motivated.

In organizations, these features are increasingly used to spark connection. Group fitness challenges, shared step goals, or collective recovery scores boost team morale and create touchpoints of collaboration, especially valuable for remote or hybrid employees who can feel isolated. When progress is tracked and celebrated together, engagement rises, and connection deepens.[20]

But remember: your data is a mirror. It reflects how you're coping, but reflection without action won't build connection. To truly shift how you feel and connect, you need to act on what the data is showing you. That's where the 'Aha Model' comes in, helping you turn awareness into habits that recharge your social battery and strengthen the relationships that fuel your wellbeing.

Your connection breakthrough

This is your turning point. With or without access to wearable data the 'Aha Model' brings together three elements to build lasting connection:

awareness, habit, and action. Together, they help you move from insight to impact, one intentional choice at a time.

Awareness: Why connection matters to you

Connection isn't an extra. It's the foundation that supports your energy, clarity, and resilience. Use this awareness exercise to tune into what connection really gives you, and why it deserves a central place in your day. That insight will fuel the habits that follow.

Pause for a moment and ask yourself:

- *When do you feel most connected, alive, and grounded?*
- *What happens to your energy, mood, and focus when you've had no meaningful connection for a few days?*
- *Which relationships (human or otherwise) make you feel safe, seen, and supported?*
- *What would change in your life if you treated connection as a daily priority rather than a nice-to-have?*

Habit: From insight to intention

Awareness is powerful but choosing *what* to do next is what transforms it. Once you've reflected on what connection gives you, it's time to turn that insight into a habit.

This doesn't mean overhauling your life. Start with one small, meaningful change that aligns with your needs. Many of my clients struggle because they prioritize what they think they *should* do, rather than the habit they *need*. Don't be tempted to connect with someone due to obligation, do so because it nourishes your soul.

Re-evaluating which connections energize you, versus those that leave you drained, creates a powerful mindset shift. You begin to prioritize your time and energy more intentionally, choosing *who* you connect with based on what truly supports your wellbeing, rather than those driven by duty or expectation.

This shift lays the foundation for deeper, healthier, and more fulfilling connections.

It starts with one question: *Which connections matter most to you right now?* Begin there.

Connection cues

- ✓ **If you're feeling lonely**: prioritize emotional closeness (e.g. a weekly call with someone who truly gets you).
- ✓ **If you're feeling flat**: prioritize energizing connection (e.g. a fun in-person catch-up with great friends).
- ✓ **If you're feeling disconnected at work**: build small bridges (e.g. start meetings with a genuine check-in or reach out to a colleague for a coffee).

Action: Embedding connection into daily life

Awareness and habit give you direction, but action locks it in. To give your connection habit an extra boost of activation energy, consider *when* you start it. Behavioural scientist Katy Milkman highlights **the fresh start effect**, the idea that you are more likely to adopt new habits when you connect them to a meaningful moment of transition.[21] These 'temporal landmarks', the start of a week, a birthday, a new season, create a psychological reset, giving you distance from the past and offering a fresh perspective on who you want to become.

These times, when you feel the potential for a new beginning, create an emotional boost that makes you more likely to take action. As Milkman's research suggests, timing your habit change around these fresh starts can make all the difference. When your new habit aligns with a fresh start, you're more likely to embrace it with energy, clarity, and intention, increasing your chances of success.

Carina experienced this first hand. Just before her 30th birthday, a milestone that prompted reflection, she committed to a wellbeing reset. That temporal landmark served as a powerful motivator, allowing her to mentally separate from old habits and embrace a new chapter focused on health and wellbeing. By aligning her goals with this fresh start, she amplified her chances of success.

The lesson is clear: timing isn't just a detail; it's a strategy. By initiating new habits during meaningful milestones, you can leverage the fresh start effect to propel yourself toward the future you envision.

Ultimately, lasting change doesn't come from grand gestures but from aligning your actions with what truly resonates. When you choose to spend time with people who energize and inspire you, not out of obligation but out of genuine desire, you naturally begin to build connections that support your wellbeing and performance.

Reflection moment

Why does your new connection habit matter to you, not just today, but long term?

What version of yourself are you choosing when you protect your time and connect for meaning, purpose, and energy?

Designing connection for modern life

Connection is a biological, emotional, and psychological pillar of performance and wellbeing underpinning how you think, feel, and perform. Prioritizing it is essential. As responsibilities expand, social circles narrow, and opportunities to meet often diminish. Being intentional about connection and investing in relationships throughout your life supports mental health and builds resilience through your network.

Across the lifespan, loneliness commonly follows a U-shaped pattern: higher in early adulthood, lowest in midlife, and rising again in older age. Social networks also tend to shrink from young adulthood onward, as time is pulled toward work and family and there are fewer built-in places to meet.[22]

Building strong relationships isn't just about maintaining old ties, it's about designing new ones. Whether you're in an open-plan office or working from your spare bedroom, connection must be created with intention. That's why designing small, regular touchpoints matters: schedule the coffees, protect the check-ins, and engage positively with your network. Resilience, creativity, and performance thrive in cultures, virtual or otherwise, where people feel seen, supported, and part of something bigger.

The strongest workplace connections grow in cultures that put human needs first, wherever you log in. Be the change maker in your workspace, shifting the social script, setting a positive tone in meetings, and building a culture that nourishes and values connection. Technology can be a powerful tool, but only when it enhances, rather than replaces, real relationships. The real opportunity lies in building a connection not based on proximity or performance, but on shared presence, intentionality, and mutual care.

As you leave this chapter, remember: the strength of your connection isn't measured by how many people you know, but by how deeply you feel seen, supported, and safe. When you feel connected, you can show up as your fullest, most energized self. That's what makes connection part of your wellbeing advantage.

Strengthen your connections

✓ **Create community spaces**: whether at work or in your neighbourhood, carve out places for genuine conversation, not just task updates.

- ✓ **Prioritize in-person interactions over passive scrolling**: swap some screen time for real connection. A coffee, a walk, or a shared meal often nourishes more than endless online interaction.
- ✓ **Choose shared activities**: walking, gardening, volunteering, or learning together. Doing something side by side strengthens bonds and reduces the pressure to 'perform' socially.
- ✓ **Expand your social network**: go beyond your immediate circle. Reach out to your colleagues, neighbours, or local community groups to strengthen resilience and belonging.
- ✓ **Value quality over quantity**: invest time with the people who help you feel safe, seen, and supported.

7

Your Sleep Habit

Let's be honest, most of us know sleep matters but don't fully appreciate just how much it underpins everything. Sleep isn't just 'switching off' at the end of the day; it's the foundation for memory, focus, energy, and emotional balance. Simply being unconscious for seven hours doesn't guarantee that your brain and body are experiencing the deep, restorative processes needed to perform, think clearly, and emotionally reset. Too often, you don't realize you're running on half-charge until illness, stress, or burnout forces you to stop.

When life is busy, sleep is often the first thing that's sacrificed. Whether it's staying up late to meet a deadline, squeezing in a workout, or just reclaiming a little personal time; sleep is pushed aside. You tell yourself you'll catch up at the weekend. That you function fine on five or six hours. I used to believe this too, until I saw the wearable data.

Before you dive into the science of sleep, it's worth pausing to ask: *How might your daily habits be shaping the quality of your sleep?*

In my coaching work I see the same pattern repeated across industries: professionals who are exhausted, but underestimate the true cost, not just physically or cognitively, but emotionally and relationally. We're living through an epidemic of tiredness. In an always-on, hyperconnected, digitally tethered culture, many of us push through the day and collapse into bed, phone in hand, hoping sleep will come.

Research confirms this disconnect. Guy Meadows, leading sleep expert and co-founder of The Sleep School, found that over 53% of adults don't know how to improve their sleep, despite reporting that poor sleep regularly affected their mood, focus, and health.[1] Many believed that lying in bed longer or catching up at the weekend would fix their fatigue.

This gap in sleep education reflects something I see in wellbeing coaching: professionals who know how to lead, present, and optimize their day, but not how to recover from it. Going to bed earlier isn't enough. Sleep isn't a light switch you turn off at night, it's a finely tuned biological rhythm. And if that rhythm is disrupted, no amount of 'catch-up sleep' can restore the clarity, calm, and energy your body is craving.

The habit that fuels all others

Sleep isn't the last step in your wellbeing journey; it's the foundation that supports everything else. When you're well-rested, you think more clearly, feel more grounded, and connect more easily with others. But when sleep is compromised, everything becomes unstable. You snap at partners, lose patience with colleagues, and start drifting from friends, not because you don't care, but because you're running on empty. Without sufficient restorative sleep, you begin to lose touch with the version of yourself you want to bring to the world.

In high-performance sport, sleep is non-negotiable. Elite athletes don't just track how hard they push; they monitor how well they recover. Increasingly, leaders are adopting the same mindset. It turns out, if you want to perform like a pro, you need to sleep like one too.

This chapter will help you reframe sleep not just as a night-time habit, but as a 24-hour rhythm that starts the moment you wake up. You'll learn how to break the 'tired but wired cycle' and calm a racing mind with simple, science-backed tools to improve your sleep tonight. And if you've ever woken after what seemed like a full night's sleep but still feel exhausted, you'll understand why. By blending neuroscience, behaviour change, and recovery strategies, this chapter will help you understand what's really going on when you sleep and how to do it better.

You're not lazy. You're not failing. You're just missing the deep, restorative sleep your brain and body need.

Meet Sofia: Tired, wired, and still showing up

Sofia is in her early 40s with two decades of experience, and a leadership role in a fast-paced tech firm. Dependable, sharp, always switched on, she's built a reputation for delivering. Like many of the professionals you meet throughout this book, Sofia doesn't realize how much this is costing her. She's exhausted and sleep is her weakest link.

Living in a buzzing city-centre apartment with her partner and their cat, Sofia keeps a full calendar. She exercises regularly, maintains a strong network, and stays on top of her responsibilities. But behind the full calendar and driven mindset, she's sliding towards burnout.

For years, she's been surviving on 5–6 hours of sleep, powered by caffeine, adrenaline, and determination. Falling asleep isn't the problem, she collapses into bed. The issue is staying asleep. Around 3:30 a.m. she jolts awake, mind racing, reaching for over-the-counter sleep aids. She tells herself this is just a phase. Something that everyone goes through as their career progresses and pressure increases. But her concentration starts slipping. She starts zoning out in meetings, forgetting details, snapping at her team. Weekends become recovery marathons, yet she never feels truly rested.

Her social life shrinks. She begins turning down plans with friends, not because she doesn't care, but because she's too tired to engage. Nights out that once energized her now feel like tasks to endure. Alcohol, which she hopes will help her unwind, only disrupts her sleep further. The spontaneity that once defined her fades.

Then comes a long-haul work trip that leaves her completely drained for weeks. Jet lag lingers, her energy flatlines, and she realizes her system isn't bouncing back. When a friend gently suggests she get support, Sofia reaches out to work with me. There's no dramatic epiphany, just an honest recognition that something needs to change.

We start small, no massive overhaul, no guilt. Just curiosity around what's really disrupting her recovery and how to introduce calm, without complexity. A wearable tracker helps her see patterns she's overlooked. Sofia begins to understand her sleep with fresh eyes. She commits to one habit change: no screens after 9 p.m.

Within weeks, her sleep scores improve. She stops waking in the early hours. Her focus returns and her mood steadies. One day during our session she pauses and says she's noticing something she hasn't felt in years: 'I feel like myself again.' It's not a dramatic revelation but it's a turning point. For Sofia, it marks the moment she realizes that prioritizing sleep isn't indulgent, it's restorative. And it's working.

Sofia's story is here to help you reflect on your own relationship with sleep and see what's possible when sleep becomes a priority. Protect your energy like it matters, because it does. Because behind every high achiever who's pushing through, there's often a nervous system begging for recovery.

Why sleep matters

Sleep is the single most powerful investment you can make for your long-term health, energy, and performance. It sharpens memory and decision-making, supports emotional regulation, strengthens the immune system, and directly influences your ability to lead, connect, and think clearly under pressure.

More than that, sleep is now recognized by researchers as a vital predictor of both healthspan and lifespan. Most adults need between seven and nine hours of quality sleep per night, not just to make it through the day, but to thrive across the decades.[2] When you invest in sleep, you invest in your lifespan.

Matthew Walker, one of the world's leading experts on sleep science, has shown that consistently sleeping fewer than six hours a night is linked to nearly every major chronic condition, including heart disease, diabetes, depression, and Alzheimer's.[3] In simple terms, the shorter your sleep, the shorter your life. If that sounds stark, it's because it is. But it's also empowering, because sleep is something you can improve, one night at a time.

High-performance sport has long recognized the critical role of sleep in recovery and performance. Many elite athletes travel with personalized pillows and mattress toppers to help optimize restorative sleep wherever they compete.[4] The data is clear: athletes who sleep fewer than seven hours a night are 1.7 times more likely to suffer injury, and up to 30% more likely to contract respiratory infections, limiting their capacity to train, compete, and recover effectively.[5]

What's true for elite athletes is just as true for you. Sleep is where your brain and body consolidate the gains of the day, whether you're preparing for a board meeting or a marathon. Without it, recovery falters, and the progress you're working so hard to achieve can stall.

Poor sleep is one of the most overlooked risk factors for burnout. It's also one of the most powerful levers for reversing it. To understand why, let's look at the sleep–stress cycle: the two-way relationship between rest and pressure and how disrupted sleep gradually fuels anxiety and burnout over time.

The sleep–stress cycle: How poor sleep fuels burnout and anxiety

Sleep and stress are locked in a two-way relationship: the more stressed you feel, the harder it is to sleep. The less you sleep, the more stressed you become. It's a cycle many professionals find themselves stuck in, one that slowly erodes energy, focus, and resilience, the very systems you rely on to perform. At the heart of this cycle is the delicate hormonal interplay between cortisol, your body's main stress hormone, and melatonin, the hormone that helps you fall and stay asleep.

In a healthy circadian rhythm, cortisol peaks naturally in the early morning to help you wake up feeling alert and ready to take on the day. As daylight fades and your body starts to wind down, cortisol drops and melatonin production increases, encouraging sleep.

But when stress is constant, the signal gets scrambled. Cortisol stays elevated well into the evening, suppressing melatonin production and delaying your natural sleep window. As a result, you feel physically exhausted but mentally alert, a state often described as 'tired but wired'.

Tired but wired

This is exactly what Sofia was experiencing. She told herself she was handling pressure well: her performance reviews were positive, her team valued her, and she was staying on top of things. But when we looked at her wearable sleep data, the story shifted. Her heart rate variability (HRV) stayed low at night. Her nervous system was still running in 'go mode' hours after work ended. Blue light from screens, late-night emails, and cycles of rumination kept cortisol high, and melatonin suppressed.

Even one hour of screen use before bed can delay melatonin release for up to 90 minutes. Watching television or scrolling may feel relaxing, but in reality, they elevate heart rate, prolong alertness, and trigger emotional activation, particularly if you fall asleep with them on.

Sofia's first step was a **digital sunset**, dimming lights and switching off screens at least 60–90 minutes before bed. Within weeks her sleep scores improved, she stopped waking in the early hours, and her energy stabilized.

It's time to uncover what's really happening while you sleep and why it starts long before your head hits the pillow. In the next section, you'll reframe sleep as part of a 24-hour rhythm, shaped by your habits from the moment you wake. This is where your circadian rhythm steps in and why understanding your weekly sleep patterns matters more than fixating on a single bad night.

Reflection moment

What does the rhythm of your evenings currently look like?

Are you giving your body a clear signal to switch off or are you dragging the stress of the day into your evening?

Sleep as a high-performance symphony

Think of your circadian rhythm like an orchestra. When all sections play in sync, light exposure, activity, nourishment, and rest, the result is harmony. But when that rhythm is disrupted by stress, late nights, irregular meals, or inconsistent routines, it's as if the conductor has lost the beat. The harmony falters. Your performance suffers.

Your night's sleep isn't one long performance from the orchestra: it's more like a symphony of movements repeating in approximately 90-minute cycles throughout the night. Each cycle carries you through distinct sleep stages, each playing a different role in restoring your body and brain. Earlier cycles in the night are dominated by deep, restorative sleep, while later cycles give more space to REM (rapid eye movement) sleep, your dream-rich phase that restores the mind.

Inside the 90-minute sleep cycle

1. **Stage 1: Light sleep (the overture)**. A brief introduction that eases your mind and body to rest. You're dozing off here. It's not long, around 5% of total sleep in adults. It sets the tone for what's to come and helps you ease into deeper sleep stages. As this is your lightest sleep stage you may easily wake, but once navigated, you transition to the next stage.
2. **Stage 2: Light-moderate sleep (the foundation)**. Your brain slows, your heart rate slows, and temperature drops as you move into a more stable rhythm. This stage consolidates memory and motor skills, laying the groundwork for sharper thinking. It accounts for around 50% of total sleep.
3. **Stage 3: Deep sleep (the power movement)**. This is your full body reset. Growth hormone surges, the immune system is reinforced, and the brain clears metabolic waste. Deep sleep typically makes up 15–25% of total sleep and is

front-loaded in the first third of your sleep period (it follows your bedtime, not the clock). If you consistently fall asleep after midnight, your deep sleep gets squeezed and recovery drops. Try nudging lights-out earlier to restore that early-night reset.

4. **REM sleep**. This is your dream sequence (the creative solo). Brain activity surges and emotional processing intensifies. It typically makes up around 20–25% of total sleep. If deep sleep restores the body, REM helps reset the emotional brain and supports insight, the 'far-apart' ideas that snap together when you wake.

The anxiety–insomnia loop

One of the most underestimated roles of sleep is its ability to restore emotional equilibrium. During REM sleep, the stage where most dreaming occurs, the brain processes and integrates emotional memories. This is why you often feel calmer and more clear-headed after a good night's sleep. It's not just physical recovery; it's a psychological reset. REM acts as your brain's emotional housekeeping system, clearing mental clutter and restoring your capacity to cope.

When sleep cycles are disrupted, you can enter the anxiety–insomnia loop. You lie awake, mind racing, replaying conversations, or worrying about what's ahead. You eventually fall asleep, but it's light and fragmented. You wake up feeling unrefreshed, anxious, and more dependent on caffeine or adrenaline to push through.

Over time the costs add up: stress tolerance drops, empathy fades, and strategic thinking narrows. You're more likely to take things personally and less able to recover from pressure or conflict. Sofia soon realized that her sleep debt wasn't just fuelling stress levels, it was eroding focus and mood across the day.

Protect your REM sleep

REM sleep increases in the final third of your sleep period, typically between 4 a.m. and 7 a.m. depending on when you fall asleep. It's the sleep stage most often lost to early alarms, shortened nights, and the anxiety–insomnia loop.

Try this tonight to optimize REM:

- ✓ **Go to bed earlier**: to protect the last part of your night.
- ✓ **Guard the final 90 minutes before sleep**: avoid alcohol, caffeine, and bright lights.
- ✓ **If an early morning is non-negotiable**: move your entire sleep window earlier rather than keeping the same bedtime and losing the REM-rich final hours.
- ✓ **If your evening runs late**: expect deep sleep to compress and REM to be the first casualty of an early alarm, then realign the following night.

Cycles not hours: Sleep lessons from high-performance sport

Sleep advice can feel confusing, but the evidence points to one clear target: most adults need 7–9 hours of sleep each night for optimal wellbeing, resilience, and cognitive performance.

Yet for those navigating demanding work, family commitments, or unpredictable schedules, consistently achieving 7–9 hours of sleep a night can feel unrealistic. A more flexible and science-backed approach comes from the world of elite sport. Instead of treating sleep as a rigid number of hours, coaches view it as a sequence of **recovery cycles**.

Nick Littlehales, sleep coach to Olympic athletes and Premier League football clubs, recommends aiming for five cycles of approximately

90 minutes per night, which equals 7.5 hours of sleep.[6] That's the ideal. But here's the powerful part: when life throws curveballs, Littlehales suggests zooming out, thinking in weekly recovery totals, and aiming for 35 sleep cycles across the week. This mindset takes the pressure off any one night and encourages you to think about recovery in rhythm, not perfection.

Instead of obsessing over a single night's missed sleep, this weekly lens lets you track your recovery more realistically amid the unpredictable demands of modern life.

Reflection moment

How many full sleep cycles are you averaging across a typical week?

What would change if you measured sleep as cycles of recovery rather than hours in bed?

Consistent sleep builds a resilient system

Aiming for 35 sleep cycles per week offers helpful breathing room; it's not a licence to burn the candle at both ends or binge recovery. It's a smarter way to build rhythm and resilience into your week when longer working hours or travel disrupts your ideal schedule. The key is still consistency.

When you try to catch up on sleep at the weekend, you often fall into what chronobiologist Till Roenneberg calls '**social jet lag**'.[7] It describes the mismatch between your body clock and your social schedule, often leaving you wide awake on Sunday night and exhausted by Tuesday morning.

Going to bed and waking at similar times (within ±60 minutes), even on weekends, helps stabilize your circadian rhythm, making it easier to fall asleep, stay asleep, and wake restored.

Energy by design: Align your day with your body clock

Not everyone is wired for early mornings. Within your circadian rhythm lies your **chronotype**, the natural timing presence that influences when you sleep, wake, and feel most alert.[8]

Chronobiology researcher Michael Breus has shown that chronotypes are largely genetic and can shape everything from sleep quality to cognitive performance and emotional resilience.[9] In short, understanding your natural rhythm can help you stop fighting your biology and start designing a lifestyle that works *with* your energy, not against it. Breus popularized the idea of four 'sleep animals': bear, lion, wolf, and dolphin, each representing a different chronotype. While not a medical diagnosis, they offer a helpful shorthand for identifying your energy patterns and personalizing your habits to match them.[10]

Reflection moment

Which sleep animal best reflects your natural rhythm?

Bear: follows the sun. Most people fall into this group. You wake and sleep easily with a mid-morning energy peak and afternoon slump. The best time for deep work is late morning.

Lion: early risers with energy that peaks in the morning. You're alert early but tend to fade by evening. Best to schedule your most important tasks before lunch.

Wolf: night animals who hit their stride in the late afternoon or evening. Mornings can feel like a slog. Late night is your zone for creative work.

Dolphin: light sleepers with erratic sleep patterns and high sensitivity to noise or stress. You may struggle with insomnia but have sharp focus mid-morning.

The reality is not everyone has full control over when they need to wake up. If your current routine doesn't match your natural rhythm, you can still make small adjustments by scheduling deep work during your natural peak hours.

For example, if you're a wolf and must wake early, you'll usually cut short late-night REM, since deep sleep clusters earlier in the night. That's why protecting total sleep time by shifting bedtime earlier when possible, and scheduling demanding work during your natural peak hours, helps preserve energy and performance, even when wake times aren't fully in your control.

Schedule lighter tasks in the morning and protect focused work for your natural peak in the afternoon or evening. Honouring your natural rhythm, even in small ways, reduces friction, makes habits easier to sustain, and protects your energy in the long term.

The trade-off behind your afternoon coffee and evening wine

You explored the impact of caffeine and alcohol in 'Your Nutrition Habit' and it's worth repeating here. While caffeine is widely used to boost energy and alcohol is often used to relax and switch off, both are among the most common sleep disruptors.

Caffeine works by blocking adenosine receptors. Adenosine builds the longer you're awake and increases your urge to sleep. When those receptors are blocked, sleepiness is masked, sleep is delayed, and natural sleep drive is blunted. Taken too late it can reduce sleep depth, and its effects can linger for up to ten hours.

It also stimulates the nervous system, which can trigger anxiety in sensitive individuals. This anxiety is one of the most common causes of insomnia, fuelling night-time rumination and a 'tired but wired' state.

Alcohol has a similar rebound effect. While it may help you fall asleep faster, it fragments your sleep and suppresses REM sleep, the stage responsible for emotional processing and creativity. That's why a late-night glass of wine can leave you groggy, flat, and irritable the next morning.

Nappuccino: The strategic nap for high performance

While caffeine is one of the most common sleep disruptors when used too late in the day, it can enhance alertness when used strategically. One proven method is the **nappuccino**, coined by cognitive neuroscientist and professor of sleep science Sara Mednick.[11] This performance-enhancing technique used by elite athletes, Formula 1 teams, and NASA pilots, pairs a short nap with caffeine for maximum effect. It's particularly effective for shift workers, long-haul travellers, and professionals facing demanding schedules who need to recover quickly.

The Nappuccino formula

1. Drink a small cup of coffee or espresso.
2. Lie down and set a timer for 20–25 minutes.
3. Wake as the caffeine takes effect, doubling the boost with alertness from the caffeine plus refreshment from the nap.

Your 24-hour sleep strategy

Sleep isn't something that just *happens* at bedtime; it's shaped by your choices all day. From the moment you wake, every choice you make from how you move, eat, rest, and connect, either builds or breaks the foundation for restorative sleep. For high performers in sport and work, poor sleep is like performing under pressure without time to recover. Over time, this hidden performance debt drains focus, erodes resilience, and weakens decision-making.

This section gives you the tools to reset the balance: simple science-backed strategies to align with your circadian rhythms, reduce stress accumulation, and create a daily routine that supports you in falling (and staying) asleep with greater ease.

Morning reset (6–9 a.m.)

The first hour of your day plays a part in whether your brain receives the right signals to wind down at night. It's why getting morning light exposure was a key component when developing your ideal morning habits.

In *Dopamine Nation*, psychiatrist and addiction specialist Anna Lembke explains how your dopamine system is easily overstimulated by screens, caffeine, sugar, and stress, leading to restlessness and reduced focus.[12] Even waiting 15 minutes before picking up your phone can serve as a powerful morning reset, stabilizing mood, reducing stress, and supporting your circadian rhythm.

Anchor your rhythm

- ✓ **Seek morning light**: step outside for 2–10 minutes within 30–60 minutes of waking, even if it's cloudy. Morning light resets your circadian clock and promotes melatonin release at night.
- ✓ **Get moving**: gentle stretching or a short walk supports your natural cortisol peak and sharpens alertness.
- ✓ **Delay screens and caffeine**: give your brain 15–30 minutes before using screens. Delay coffee by 60–90 minutes to allow cortisol to peak naturally.

Midday management (1–3 p.m.)

Your body naturally experiences a drop in alertness after lunch. This isn't a sign of laziness, it's biology. Known as the post-lunch dip, it's part of your circadian rhythm, a predictable low point in your energy cycle that typically occurs between 1 p.m. and 3 p.m. In elite sport this is known as your **recovery window**. It's a time when rest, light movement, or short naps can support physical and cognitive regeneration.

In most workplaces this dip is ignored or powered through for another productivity sprint. It's often masked with caffeine which only delays melatonin release and makes it harder to switch off later.

Protect your afternoon dip

✓ **Reset with rest**: take a 5–10 minute pause for guided breathwork or a mindful walk to downshift stress and restore focus.

✓ **Experiment with a 'nappuccino'**: as long as it's practised before 2 p.m. it won't harm your night's sleep.

✓ **Avoid caffeine after 2 p.m.**: late-day stimulants reduce deep sleep and fragment recovery.

Evening wind-down (8–10 p.m.)

Falling asleep is a *dimmer*, not a switch. Melatonin, the hormone that helps you fall asleep, is released in response to darkness and calm. But scrolling social media, answering messages, or watching high stimulus content sends the opposite signal: stay alert. Matthew Walker calls this the '**cognitive second wind**', a burst of brain activity fuelled by artificial light and digital noise.[13]

Blue light, especially from screens, suppresses melatonin. When your brain perceives blue light, it assumes it's daytime and delays the natural sleep process.[14] If screen use is necessary, use night mode, blue light-blocking glasses, or shift to audio-based content to reduce visual stimulation.

How to sleep like a pro even at 3 a.m.

Waking in the middle of the night isn't failure, it's normal. In fact, brief awakenings happen naturally at the end of every 90-minute sleep cycle. Most will pass unnoticed, but they can feel disruptive, especially in midlife when sleep becomes lighter.

Many of my clients worry they're somehow *bad* at sleeping if they're awake at 3 a.m. But here's the truth: if you're asleep for 80–85% of your time in bed, that's considered restorative. What matters most is how you respond if you wake in the night.

Temperature plays a vital role in sleep. Your body needs to cool slightly to drift into deeper sleep. When you're too warm, which may be due to hormonal changes, this cooling is disrupted and night-time wakings become more common. Perimenopause can interfere with temperature regulation, leaving many women frustrated by restless nights.

Practical strategies to work with your body include a warm, not hot, shower before bed to lower core temperature by drawing heat to the surface of the skin. If you share a bed, using separate duvets allows each person to regulate their heat without disturbing the other. Choosing breathable fabrics such as cotton, bamboo, or linen, instead of synthetics that trap heat can create a cooler, more comfortable environment.

Avoid the wide-awake club

- ✓ **Don't check your clock**: checking the time can trigger mental alertness and sleep-related stress. Calm reassurance helps your brain stay in sleep mode.
- ✓ **If wakeful after 20–30 minutes**: get up, keep lights low, and do a quiet relaxing activity (reading, or listening to soft music). Return to bed when drowsy.
- ✓ **Shift your focus to rest**: don't try to force sleep. Quiet rest is still restorative, even if it's not unconscious sleep.

What your wearable tells you about Your Sleep Habit

Your sleep data is more than a tally of hours. It reveals how well your body is recovering, how deep your sleep truly is, and whether your habits, especially at the end of the day, are helping or hindering your restoration. Sleep isn't just about duration, it's about depth, rhythm, and consistency.

Of all the available wearable metrics, many of my clients feel swamped by sleep data. The graphs, acronyms, and scores tell them their sleep is poor without explaining what to do next. As always, the real value lies in spotting trends over time and not obsessing over a single bad night. When interpreted well, your wearable can help you understand not only *how* you're sleeping, but *why* your sleep might be disrupted and *what* to do to get it back on track.

Sleep score

This is a combined score reflecting your overall recovery through sleep based on duration, depth, restlessness, and timing, usually shown out of 100. You'll often see your sleep duration displayed as a raw number alongside a breakdown of the night. While most adults typically need at least seven hours of sleep for optimal functioning, don't panic if your wearable shows six hours occasionally. It's the weekly pattern that matters more than a single night.

What to look for:

- **Scores in the 80s or higher**: usually suggest solid, restorative sleep.
- **Scores in the 60s or below**: often reflect disrupted rhythms, stress, or environmental factors. Your body is sending a signal to reset.

Sleep stages (light, deep, REM)

Many wearables break your night into sleep stages based on HRV, movement, and in some cases skin temperature. These are estimates, not direct measures of brain activity which means the patterns don't always reflect the typical 90-minute cycle described earlier in the chapter. Your device can't diagnose sleep disorders or capture the full complexity of sleep, but it can help you spot trends that highlight how your habits and lifestyle influence recovery.

When your wearable reports something like REM: 20%, that number refers to the percentage of your total sleep time spent in that specific stage. It's not a direct measure of quality, but it helps you see which stages are getting squeezed. Generally, sleep earlier in the night supports more physical recovery, while longer sleep duration contributes to deeper mental and emotional restoration.

What to look for:

- **Light sleep (50–60%)**: this accounts for the bulk of your night. This stage supports essential functions including learning and memory.
- **Deep sleep (15–25%)**: this is critical for physical recovery, immune health, and body repair.
- **REM sleep (20–25%)**: this supports mood, memory, and emotional processing.
- **Consistently low deep or REM sleep**: this may reflect stress, caffeine, alcohol, or inconsistent sleep timing. Use this as a signal to review your evening habits.

Sleep efficiency

Sleep efficiency reflects how effectively you sleep once you're in bed. It's calculated as the percentage of time asleep compared with total time in bed. A healthy range is 80–85%. If your efficiency dips below 75%, the solution isn't simply more time in bed, it's about improving your wind-down routines.

What to look for:

- **Efficiency below 75%:** lying in bed longer usually backfires. Instead review relaxation habits or shorten your sleep window to match actual sleep time.
- **Drops after stressful evenings:** notice how overstimulation (screen, alcohol, late work) often reduces efficiency.
- **Higher efficiency on calmer days:** this is a positive sign your overall balance and evening routine are supporting better sleep.

Daily readiness score

Sleep has been described as the greatest legal performance-enhancing drug.[15] Your readiness score gives you a daily, personalized glimpse of just how much that performance-enhancing drug is working for or against you.

What to look for:

- **Scores of 85–100:** this is a sign of optimal readiness. You're well recovered and ready to perform at your best.
- **Scores of 70–84:** this shows good readiness. You're functioning well but could benefit from more consistency in sleep, rest, or recovery habits.
- **Scores of 60–69:** this is the watchful zone. Use this as a signal to adjust workload, focus on hydration, or add extra recovery.
- **Consistently 60 or below:** this may reflect elevated stress, disrupted sleep, or chronic under-recovery. Use this as a prompt to reset.

Reflection moment

What does your wearable say about your sleep and how does it compare to how you feel?

Are you using your data to adjust and restore, or just to confirm you're tired?

Heart rate variability

A key indicator of nervous system balance, HRV is not a sleep score. As a core metric it helps complete the picture of whether your body is adapting well or under strain. By highlighting shifts in strain and recovery, HRV helps you understand when it may be time to adjust your sleep and recovery habits.

What to look for:

- **Dips after poor sleep or stressful evenings**: this suggests your body isn't getting the restorative sleep it needs.
- **Rises after deep, consistent sleep**: this typically reflects better stress resilience and recovery capacity.
- **Your personal baseline**: HRV is highly individual; look at your own trends over time, not comparisons with others.

Sofia's wearable insights

When Sofia explores her wearable data with me for the first time she's curious and a little sceptical. Like many of my clients, she didn't think she had a sleep problem. She was tired, sure, but assumed that was just part of being successful, busy, and driven. 'I fall asleep fast,' she said, 'and I'm in bed by 11 p.m. most nights so I must be doing okay'. But the data suggested otherwise.

When she first tracks her sleep, she notices HRV dipping after late-evening emails or a glass or two of red wine. Readiness lingers in the 50s despite enough hours in bed, and sleep efficiency often sits below 75%. She was in bed, but her body wasn't *recovering*.

For Sofia, a shift in her sleep quality didn't happen just because she slept longer. It happened when she started making small, consistent changes to her routine. By getting outside for morning light, dropping her mid-week glasses of wine, and committing to an earlier wind-down, her HRV trends, readiness and sleep scores begin to rise. The connection between actions and metrics doesn't just inform her; it gives her direction and momentum.

Sofia didn't need to overhaul her life, just make smarter choices with her biology in mind. When clients like Sofia see their sleep patterns reflected in a clear, supportive way without judgement, they begin to understand what their body's been trying to say all along. The data stops being abstract and becomes practical.

Wearable insights don't just help you sleep better. They help you live with energy, clarity, and capacity you didn't realize you were missing. Not everyone uses wearable technology and that's okay. Your body already provides daily clues about your sleep; the key is learning to notice and interpret them.

Your sleep breakthrough

When it comes to improving sleep, it's easy to feel swamped by expert tips and online hacks, as if you need to fix everything. You don't. Start by pausing, reflecting, and identifying the one change that matters most to you. Maybe it's setting a wind-down routine, reducing evening screen time, or noticing how caffeine impacts your sleep quality. One shift to your routine can unlock a new level of energy, clarity, and rest. This is where the 'Aha Model' comes in.

Awareness: Reframe your relationships with sleep

The most powerful breakthrough happens when you start to view sleep differently. Reframe your understanding of sleep as a 24-hour rhythm, not just the hours you're asleep. Notice how your habits throughout the day, from getting more daylight, to taking breaks in the afternoon and ending with a calm evening routine, shape what your body can do while you sleep. Raise your awareness by observing the moments you pause, breathe, and intentionally build restorative practice into your day.

- *Do you regularly get natural light within the first hour of waking?*
- *What time do you typically have your last caffeinated drink?*

- *What are your wind-down habits in the hour before bed, and how well are they serving you? Screens off, dimmed lighting, relaxation, or are you still working, checking email, and watching a gripping TV series?*

Habit: Find the sleep habit that works for you

Sleep can be tricky as it's influenced by countless variables, from stress and light exposure to nutrition and hormones. That's why personalized sleep habits matter.

Whether it's a morning walk, setting a caffeine cut-off, or protecting a consistent bedtime, choose one action that feels doable and meaningful. Small changes build big results, especially when repeated.

Reflection moment

Which one of the following wellbeing habits: routine, movement, nutrition, balance, rest, or connection, would improve tonight's sleep if you gave it just 10% more attention?

Action: Habits in the Goldilocks zone

One of the biggest barriers to sustaining new habits isn't effort, it's motivation. Motivation fluctuates and that's normal. You lose momentum when a habit feels either too hard or too easy. That's where James Clear's '**The Goldilocks Rule**' helps you find the middle ground; you're more likely to stick with a new habit when the challenge is just right; not too difficult, not too easy, just right.[16]

When it comes to building your sleep habit, that means choosing an action you can keep even on your busiest day. Instead of giving up caffeine entirely, set a consistent 2 p.m. caffeine cut-off. Rather than chasing a perfect bedtime, protect a 30-minute wind-down with lights dimmed and screens off. These small, repeatable wins keep your brain engaged and nudge you towards what psychologists call a *flow state*: the feeling of being fully immersed in something, focused, absorbed, and progressing.

When motivation dips, reduce to your minimum viable habit; five minutes of wind-down still counts. Use prompts to help make the habit automatic. If you miss a day, forgive fast and resume fast.

The real difference between long-term success and burnout isn't how hard you push when you're energized, it's what you do when the habit feels repetitive, inconvenient, or hard. Anyone can show up when they feel motivated. Sticking to your habit on the days you feel tired, distracted, or over it is the difference between dabbling in wellbeing and making real progress.

Reflection moment

What habit feels 'just right' for this week, challenging enough to matter, but not so hard you'll abandon it? What is your minimum version of that habit for low-energy days?

The habit that fuels all others

Let's be clear, sleep isn't just one of the seven wellbeing habits; it's the keystone that stabilizes every other habit. It restores your energy for movement, sharpens your thinking for routine, strengthens your emotional resilience for connection, and helps you make better decisions around nutrition, balance, and rest. Without quality sleep, every other habit becomes harder to sustain. When sleep is protected, everything else gets easier.

Yet most of us try to push through. We ignore the signs, normalize tiredness, and tell ourselves that 'just a couple of glasses of wine' or 'just one late night' won't matter. As Sofia discovered, real breakthrough doesn't require a complete overhaul. It starts with consistent habit change and honest reflection. When she looked at her data, working late, replying to emails with a glass of wine in hand, she saw the cost. Her awareness was raised; real change began.

Your own breakthrough may come through wearable insights, or through a feeling, sense, or realization that something needs to shift. With one cue, one habit, one decision, you can protect your sleep, not as an afterthought, but as a non-negotiable part of who you are.

This chapter hasn't been about sleep perfection; it's about sleep protection. Recognize the patterns, reclaim your natural rhythm, and realize that small daily changes, like dimming lights, stepping outside first thing, or closing the laptop an hour earlier, have a far bigger impact than most people realize. You don't need to change everything. You just need to do one thing differently tonight. Every night is an opportunity to begin again, calmly, clearly, and with the intention to make one change and repeat it.

Build your sleep routine

- ✓ **Seek sunlight early**: step outside within 30 minutes of waking, even if it's cloudy. Morning light anchors your circadian clock, promoting melatonin release at night.
- ✓ **Set a caffeine cut-off**: aim to avoid caffeine after 2 p.m. to protect deep sleep and reduce sleep latency.
- ✓ **Use the 3-2-1 rule**: no food 3 hours before bed, no fluids 2 hours before, no screens 1 hour before.
- ✓ **Create a sleep cue**: dim lights, light yoga to unwind, journal, or listen to music to signal 'powering down'.
- ✓ **Digital sunset**: switch off devices at least 60–90 minutes before bed to minimize melatonin suppression.
- ✓ **Be consistent**: keep regular bed and wake times, even at weekends, so your body can predict and optimize sleep.

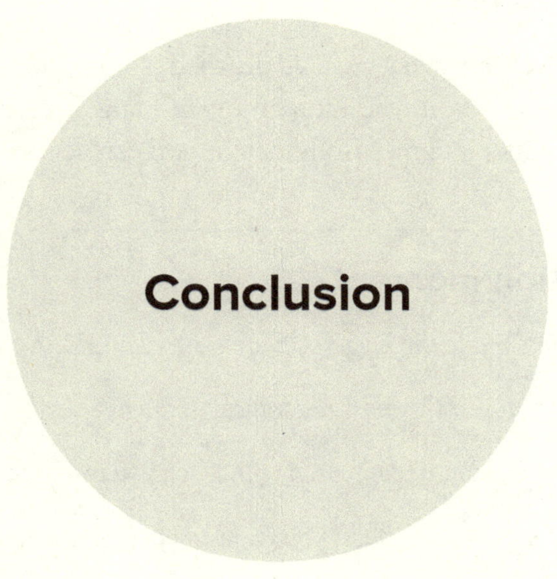

Conclusion

Congratulations! You've been prioritizing yourself in a world that constantly pulls your attention elsewhere. Reading this book wasn't just about learning new strategies, it was an act of intention. You've paused, reflected, and taken meaningful action.

You've also made space in your day for something that often gets pushed aside: your health, clarity, and energy. That matters because the way you feel fuels how you live, lead, and connect.

Through these pages, you've explored seven transformative habits, each one backed by science, grounded in real life, and designed to help you feel better, think clearly, and perform at your best. Together, they create a foundation that will continue to support you long after the book closes.

More importantly, you've begun to shift your identity. You're no longer someone trying to be healthy, you're becoming someone who puts wellbeing at the heart of how they live. It's not something you do; it's part of who you are.

Review and reset

Pause to reflect on what you've learned so far, because without reviewing progress you lose momentum. Change doesn't come from information alone; it comes from insight you can act on.

Reflection moment

Which habits made the biggest difference to your day?

Where did you feel the most resistance, and why?

How do you feel today, compared with when you began this journey?

What's the number one habit you want to hold on to and build from here?

Here's the truth: if you don't protect your energy, you lose it. If you don't prioritize recovery, you stay stuck in survival mode and drift toward compromised wellbeing and the risk of burnout. You don't need to change everything. Just focus on the habit that matters most, then build from there.

Wellbeing as a framework for life

Even with the best tools and the greatest will in the world, real life can get in the way. You'll miss a day, feel stretched, and lose momentum. This is absolutely part of the process and must never be seen as failure.

Sustainable wellbeing isn't about perfection. It's about consistency. The science of behaviour change shows setbacks are normal, and with the right mindset they become stepping stones.

Making wellbeing last

- ✓ **Track your progress**: insight builds momentum.
- ✓ **Design flexible habits**: personalize to your life and adapt as your circumstances change.
- ✓ **Build a wellbeing identity**: it's part of who you are.
- ✓ **Stay connected with others**: wellbeing thrives in company.
- ✓ **Celebrate your progress**: small wins fuel long-term momentum.
- ✓ **Keep learning and adjusting**: this is an ongoing journey, not the finish line.

Next steps

Your wellbeing is your most valuable asset. Protect it, nurture it, and watch how every part of your life transforms. As you continue to practise the seven transformative habits remember that the true advantage begins when action meets intention. This is where knowledge creates change and habit becomes identity.

Your wellbeing is the foundation that enables you to show up fully, bringing your best self to work and home again. The real advantage begins as you journey from knowing what works, into living it.

This is your time to thrive.

Living *The Wellbeing Advantage*

1. **The Routine Habit**: start your day with energy and focus by creating consistent mornings that align with your natural rhythms. Notice how your readiness score or morning energy check reflects these changes.
2. **The Movement Habit**: build vitality and strength by weaving activity into your daily life. Use wearable feedback, like resting heart rate (RHR), or simple self-checks to guide when to push and when to pause.
3. **The Nutrition Habit**: stabilize energy and sharpen thinking with simple nutrition and hydration strategies. Track how changes affect focus, mood, and your body's daily readiness.
4. **The Balance Habit**: balance ambition with capacity. Prioritize, set boundaries, and use wearable data or a weekly self-check to adjust commitments up or down as needed.
5. **The Rest Habit**: recharge with micro-breaks. See how even short recovery moments shift stress load or notice the clear-headed lift they bring.
6. **The Connection Habit**: strengthen relationships that buffer stress and boost resilience. Pay attention to how quality connection improves mood, recovery, and energy.
7. **The Sleep Habit**: restore your energy with deeper, more consistent sleep. Your wearable may highlight improvements in sleep stages and recovery, but what you'll notice is clearer focus, and steadier energy that carries through the day.

Glossary

Adenosine A chemical in the brain that builds up while you are awake and creates sleep pressure. It clears during deep sleep, helping you feel refreshed.

Autonomic nervous system The body's automatic control system that regulates heart rate, breathing, digestion, and stress responses. It includes the sympathetic ('fight or flight') and parasympathetic ('rest and digest') branches.

Body battery A simple way to describe the energy you have available. It's influenced by rest, nutrition, movement, and stress. When your body battery is high, you feel well-rested and ready to take on demands; when it's low, even small tasks feel draining. Managing it means balancing activity with recovery.

Burnout A state of physical, emotional, and mental exhaustion that builds up when stress is prolonged and recovery is missing. It often shows up as constant fatigue, reduced motivation, and a sense of detachment from work. Burnout isn't a personal failing; it's a signal that the balance between demands and resources needs to be restored.

Circadian rhythm Your body's internal 24-hour clock that regulates when you feel awake, alert, or sleepy. Controlled by the brain, it influences energy, mood, hormone release, digestion, and sleep–wake patterns. Light exposure is the strongest cue for keeping your circadian rhythm on track.

Cortisol A hormone produced by the adrenal glands in response to stress. Often called the 'stress hormone', it helps manage energy, regulate blood sugar, support metabolism, and control inflammation. While short bursts of cortisol can be helpful (e.g. increasing alertness in a high-pressure situation), chronically elevated cortisol, often linked to ongoing stress, poor sleep, or poor nutrition, can contribute to fatigue, irritability, weight gain, and lowered immunity.

Deep sleep The most physically restorative stage of sleep. Typically concentrated in the first half of the night; supports tissue repair, aspects of memory, and immune function. Deep sleep helps you wake feeling refreshed and recharged the next day.

Dopamine A neurotransmitter involved in motivation, reward, learning, and movement. It rises when you anticipate or achieve something rewarding which helps reinforce habits. Brief, moderate spikes are useful for focus and drive; chronic high stimulation can dull sensitivity over time, making it harder to feel satisfied. Steady routines help keep dopamine responses balanced.

Heart rate variability (HRV) The tiny differences in time between your heartbeats, measured in milliseconds. Higher HRV generally indicates greater adaptability and resilience to stress; lower HRV can signal fatigue, stress, or insufficient recovery. Track trends over time (not single days) to understand how well your nervous system is balancing stress and rest.

Melatonin A hormone produced by the pineal gland in the brain, released primarily in darkness. Melatonin helps synchronize your circadian rhythm and signals 'biological night', promoting sleep onset and supporting sleep timing. Evening bright light can suppress melatonin and delay sleep while consistent morning light helps keep its daily rhythm on track.

Parasympathetic nervous system The 'rest and digest' branch of the autonomic nervous system. It slows heart rate, supports digestion, and promotes recovery after stress. Practices such as controlled breathing, gentle movement, or mindful pauses can help engage parasympathetic activity.

Readiness score A daily indicator provided by some wearables that combines data such as heart rate variability (HRV), resting heart rate (RHR), sleep quality, and recovery to summarize how prepared your body is to handle stress or activity. A higher score suggests you have the capacity to push ahead, while a lower score signals it's time to prioritize recovery.

Real-time heart rate Your current heart rate shown live on a wearable device or measured manually by checking your pulse at points like the wrist or neck. It reflects your immediate activity level, stress, or recovery state, helping you notice how daily events affect your body.

REM sleep A sleep stage associated with vivid dreaming, emotional processing, and aspects of learning and creativity. During rapid eye movement (REM) sleep, the brain is highly active while the body remains largely still.

Resting heart rate (RHR) The number of times your heart beats per minute when you're at complete rest. A lower RHR often indicates better cardiovascular fitness and recovery; a higher RHR can signal stress, fatigue, or illness. Tracking RHR over time helps you spot meaningful changes in your health and recovery.

Serotonin A neurotransmitter that supports mood, motivation, appetite, and the sleep–wake cycle. Daylight exposure, movement, and social connection can help optimize serotonin levels. Serotonin is also a precursor for melatonin, the hormone that signals your body it's time to sleep.

Social battery A way to describe the energy you have available for social interaction. Some people recharge through connection; others feel drained by too much of it. Protecting and recharging your social battery means knowing your limits and finding the right balance of solitude and connection.

Sympathetic nervous system The branch of your nervous system that activates the 'fight-or-flight' response. It raises heart rate and sharpens focus to prepare you for challenge. While essential in short bursts, if the sympathetic system stays dominant for too long it can drain energy, disrupt sleep, and impact long-term wellbeing.

Further reading

Introduction

Attia, P., & Gifford, B. (2023). *Outlive: the science and art of longevity*. Harmony Books.

Clear, J. (2018). *Atomic habits: an easy and proven way to build good habits and break bad ones*. Avery.

Duhigg, C. (2012). *The power of habit: why we do what we do in life and business*. Random House.

1 Your Routine Habit

Fogg, B. J. (2020). *Tiny habits: the small changes that change everything*. Houghton Mifflin Harcourt.

Fredrickson, B. L. (2009). *Positivity: groundbreaking research to release your inner optimist and thrive*. Crown Publishers.

Walker, M. (2017). *Why we sleep: unlocking the power of sleep and dreams*. Penguin Books.

2 Your Movement Habit

Achor, S. (2010). *The happiness advantage: the seven principles of positive psychology that fuel success and performance at work*. Crown Business.

Lieberman, D. (2021). *Exercised: the science of physical activity, rest and health*. Penguin Books.

McGonigal, K. (2019). *The joy of movement: how exercise helps us find happiness, hope, connection, and courage*. Avery.

3 Your Nutrition Habit

Philpotts, R. (2023). *The burnout bible*. Practical Inspiration.

Spector, T. (2015). *The diet myth: the real science behind what we eat*. Weidenfeld and Nicolson.

van Tulleken, C. (2023). *Ultra-processed people: why do we all eat stuff that isn't food and why can't we stop?* Cornerstone Press.

4 Your Balance Habit

Dweck, C. S. (2006). *Mindset: the new psychology of success*. Random House.

Nagoski, E., & Nagoski, A. (2019). *Burnout: the secret to unlocking the stress cycle*. Ballantine Books.

Wood, W. (2019). *Good habits, bad habits: the science of making positive changes that stick*. Macmillan Business.

5 Your Rest Habit

Chatterjee, R. (2018). *The stress solution: the 4 steps to reset your body, mind, relationships and purpose*. Penguin Life.

Dalton-Smith, S. (2017). *Sacred rest: recover your life, renew your energy, restore your sanity*. Faith Words.

Hammond, C. (2019). *The art of rest: how to find respite in the modern age*. Canongate Books.

6 Your Connection Habit

Achor, S. (2013). *Before happiness: the 5 hidden keys to achieving success, spreading happiness, and sustaining positive change*. Crown Business.

Chatterjee, R. (2022). *Happy mind, happy life: 10 simple ways to feel great every day*. Penguin Life.

Murthy, V. H. (2020). *Together: the healing power of human connection in a sometimes lonely world*. Harper Wave.

7 Your Sleep Habit

Foster, R. (2022). *Life time: the new science of the body clock and how it can revolutionize your sleep and health*. Penguin Life.

Lembke, A. (2021). *Dopamine nation: finding balance in the age of indulgence*. Dutton.

Littlehales, N. (2016). *Sleep: the myth of 8 hours, the power of naps and the new plan to recharge your body and mind*. Penguin Life.

Walker, M. (2017). *Why we sleep: unlocking the power of sleep and dreams*. Scribner.

Acknowledgements

Gratitude, before anything else. This book may be written by me, but it was supported by many hands; life as it turns out, is a team sport. I wrote with the long view in mind: to maximize healthspan so I can enjoy the everyday moments and the milestones with my boys, Toby and Max, watching them grow, dream, and fly, and one day share these habits with families of their own.

First and foremost, my love and thanks to my husband, Ken. In life, as in work, you stand with me, steady, encouraging, and generous with the space and time for ideas to form and sentences to land. Before long, a book is born. Thank you. Now, get on your bike and plot the next adventure, with a few more habits to help it go the distance.

How can we help? My family ask this often and mean it. My parents' positivity and support have long given me the confidence to pursue my ambitions; thanks for always believing in me. Elder (and she insists wiser) sister Sarah has been cheerleading from the first word, nudging me toward writing retreats (we'll get there one day sis, Gerry will hold the fort)! My brother Louis and my sister-in-law/walking-buddy Laura: your resilience is the benchmark I strive toward. To the van Someren family cheering from afar, thank you. Family: always there, always supporting.

I'm blessed with kind, funny, fiercely supportive friends. Lucy, Vicks, Sarah, Charlotte, Aoife, Vu, Karen, Sarah, Lewis, Joe and Aoife, thank you for the check-ins, the voice notes, your faith in me. I don't take it lightly. A special shout-out to Vivienne and Zoe, your support genuinely shifted my life and career trajectory; thanks for making the harder parts lighter. Lisa, Eilish, Katie, and Carol, your positivity, curiosity, and interest from the first spark were the activation energy that kept me going in those early days.

To my Wellbeing Trailblazers crew, especially Cepta, Laura, and Bridget, thank you for showing up to share, explore, and solve wellbeing challenges. To my clients, past and present, thank you for trusting me with your stories. You inspire the tools in these pages, and any clarity here comes from walking alongside you. When Adrian Kelly introduced me to my inspirational publisher, Alison Jones, at his book launch, I didn't imagine I'd be writing my own book within three months. Thanks Adrian, for your continued support, and thank you to the wonderful PIP team and the authors I've met along the way. I can't wait to read what we bring into the world!

To ex-colleagues, early readers, and kind endorsers who believed in my book before there was a cover! Bernadette Dancy, Sophia Hodges, Sharon Fitzmaurice, and Clare McKenna to name but a few, thank you.

I opened with gratitude, and I'll close with the same; some habits are worth keeping! Gratitude for the friends and family who supported me, and for you, the reader who gives the most precious commodity: your time. I hope you feel supported, seen, and energized to make the small changes that matter most, so you can enjoy a longer, fuller life with the people you love. That is, after all, the point of all of this.

About the author

Dr Janine van Someren translates high-performance science into everyday wellbeing, showing professionals how to thrive without burning out. Drawing on more than 25 years' experience across sport, academia, and corporate consulting, she brings a rare mix of scientific expertise and real-world practicality to the challenges of modern working life.

Her expertise is underpinned by a PhD in Life Story Research and a Master's in Applied Human Science. Her doctoral work uncovered how the high-performance habits of elite women tennis players at Wimbledon can be adapted for life beyond the court, laying the foundations of transformative habits across a lifetime.

Janine founded 'The Wellbeing Advantage', a consultancy delivering programmes for Fortune 500 companies and Fortune Global 500 organizations, including NASDAQ, Stryker, and Unilever. Her insights on stress, recovery, and resilience have been featured on RTÉ Radio, *The Business Post*, and Newstalk's *Alive and Kicking*. As a sought-after speaker and podcast guest, she is known for turning complex evidence into clear, usable tools on topics spanning hybrid work, women's health, and the future of wellbeing in an AI-enabled world.

Alongside her corporate work, Janine supports clients one-to-one with navigating career change, midlife transitions, or returning to work after serious illness. Having walked the road herself, she combines expertise with genuine empathy to help clients regain clarity, rebuild confidence, and restore energy. Grounded in science yet human at its core, her work empowers people to move beyond burnout and design lives that sustain both performance and wellbeing.

To find out more visit https://thewellbeingadvantage.com

Notes and references

Introduction

1 Mental Health UK. (2025). *The burnout report January 2025*. https://mentalhealth-uk.org/burnout
2 Attia, P., & Gifford, B. (2023). *Outlive: the science and art of longevity*. Vermilion.
3 Diener, E., & Chan, M. Y. (2011). Happy people live longer: subjective well-being contributes to health and longevity. *Applied Psychology: Health and Well-Being*, 3(1), 1–43. https://doi.org/10.1111/j.1758-0854.2010.01045.x
4 Deloitte. (2025). *Digital consumer trends 2025*. Also found that smartwatch access has risen from 28% in 2023 to 33% in 2025. https://www.deloitte.com/uk/en/Industries/tmt/research/digital-consumer-trends.html
5 Ledger, D., & McCaffrey, D. (2022). *Inside wearables: how the science of human behaviour change offers the secret to long-term engagement*. Endeavour Partners.
6 Van der Kolk, B. (2014). *The body keeps the score: brain, mind, and body in the healing of trauma*. Penguin.
7 Huberman is best known for translating neuroscience into practical, evidence-based tools. He is the host of *Huberman Lab Podcast*; episodes can be accessed here: www.hubermanlab.com/podcast

1 Your Routine Habit

1 Brooks, A. W., Schroeder, J., Risen, J. L., Gino, F., Galinsky, A. D., Norton, M. I., & Schweitzer, M. E. (2016). Don't stop believing: Rituals improve performance by decreasing anxiety. *Organizational Behavior and Human Decision Processes*, 137, 71–85. https://doi.org/10.1016/j.obhdp.2016.07.004

2 McEwen, B. S. (1998). Protective and damaging effects of stress mediators. *New England Journal of Medicine*, 338(3), 171–179. https://doi.org/10.1056/NEJM199801153380307

3 Moss, J. (2021). Beyond burned out. *Harvard Business Review*, 99(2), 38–47. https://hbr.org/2021/02/beyond-burned-out

4 Discover more about micro-stress doses in Chatterjee, R. (2018). *The stress solution: the 4 steps to reset your body, mind, relationships and purpose.* Penguin Life.

5 Huberman, A. (2022). Using light to optimize health. *Huberman Lab Podcast.* www.hubermanlab.com/episode/using-light-sunlight-blue-light-and-red-light-to-optimize-health

6 Walker, M. (2017). *Why we sleep: the new science of sleep and dreams.* Penguin Books.

7 Rozentals, A. (2023). Starting your day checking email is counterproductive. *Forbes*, 10 August. www.forbes.com/councils/forbesbusinesscouncil/2023/08/10/starting-your-day-checking-email-is-counterproductive/

8 Vohs, K. D., Baumeister, R. F., Schmeichel, B. J., Twenge, J. M., Nelson, N. M., & Tice, D. M. (2008). Making choices impairs subsequent self-control: A limited-resource account of decision making, self-regulation, and active initiative. *Journal of Personality and Social Psychology*, 94(5), 883–898. https://doi.org/10.1037%2F0022-3514.94.5.883

9 Fogg, B. J. (2020). *Tiny habits: the small changes that change everything.* Houghton Mifflin Harcourt.

10 Duhigg, C. (2012). *The power of habit: why we do what we do in life and business.* Random House. Duhigg is a Pulitzer Prize-winning journalist and author, best known for translating behavioural science research into practical strategies for habit formation, productivity, and decision-making.

11 Stickgold, R., Malia, A., Maguire, D., Roddenberry, D., & O'Connor, M. (2000). Replaying the game: hypnagogic images in normals and amnesics. *Science*, 290(5490), 350–353. https://doi.org/10.1126/science.290.5490.350

12 Achor, S. (2010). *The happiness advantage: the seven principles of positive psychology that fuel success and performance at work*. Crown Business.

13 Emmons, R. A. (2007). *Thanks! How the new science of gratitude can make you happier*. Houghton Mifflin.

14 Professor Wendy Wood's research shows that most of our actions are automatic, shaped by repetition and environment, not willpower. In her book *Good habits, bad habits*, she explains how effective change doesn't come from trying harder, but from designing systems that support consistent, low-effort habits. Wood, W. (2019). *Good habits, bad habits: the science of making positive changes that stick*. Macmillan Business.

15 Brecheisen, J. (2023). Flexible work is having a mixed impact on employee well-being and productivity. *Harvard Business Review*, 16 October. https://hbr.org/2023/10/research-flexible-work-is-having-a-mixed-impact-on-employee-well-being-and-productivity

16 Barbara Fredrickson is a leading researcher in positive psychology, best known for her 'Broaden-and-Build Theory' of positive emotions. In her book *Positivity*, she explores how cultivating small, frequent moments of positivity, such as mindfulness, movement, and connection, can build emotional resilience, lower stress, and enhance overall wellbeing over time. Fredrickson, B. L. (2009). *Positivity: top-notch research reveals the 3-to-1 ratio that will change your life*. Crown Archetype.

17 Lally, P., van Jaarsveld, C. H. M., Potts, H. W. W., & Wardle, J. (2009). How are habits formed: modelling habit formation in the real world. *European Journal of Social Psychology*, 40(6), 998–1009. https://doi.org/10.1002/ejsp.674

18 Wood, W. (2019). *Good habits, bad habits: the science of making positive changes that stick*. Macmillan Business.

19 Fredrickson, B. L. (2001). The role of positive emotions in positive psychology: the broaden-and-build theory of positive emotions. *American Psychologist*, 56(3), 218–226. https://doi.org/10.1037%2F0003-066X.56.3.218

2 Your Movement Habit

1 Lieberman, D. (2021). *Exercised: the science of physical activity, rest and health*. Penguin Books.

2 McGonigal, K. (2019). *The joy of movement: how exercise helps us find happiness, hope, connection, and courage*. Avery.

3 Ekelund, U., Tarp, J., Steene-Johannessen, J., Hansen, B. H., Jefferis, B., Fagerland, M. W., Whincup, P., Diaz, K. M., Hooker, S. P., Chernofsky, A., Larson, M. G., Spartano, N. L., Vasan, R. S., Dohrn, I.-M., Hagströmer, M., Edwardson, C., Yates, T., Shiroma, E., Anderssen, S. A., & Lee, I.-M. (2019). Dose-response associations between accelerometery measured physical activity and sedentary time and all-cause mortality: Systematic review and harmonised meta-analysis. *British Medical Journal*, 366, l4570. www.bmj.com/content/366/bmj.l4570

4 The concept of GAS was first proposed by Hans Selye in 1950. Selye, H. (1950). Stress and the general adaptation syndrome. *British Medical Journal*, 1(4667), 1383–1392. www.bmj.com/content/1/4667/1383

More recent developments in stress science, including Bruce McEwen's work on allostatic load: McEwen, B. S. (1998). Protective and damaging effects of stress mediators. *New England Journal of Medicine*, 338(3), 171–179. https://doi.org/10.1056/NEJM199801153380307; and Robert Sapolsky's research on chronic stress, have expanded our understanding of how prolonged stress impacts physical and mental health. Sapolsky, R. M. (2004). *Why zebras don't get ulcers: the acclaimed guide to stress, stress-related diseases, and coping* (3rd ed.). Henry Holt and Company.

5 Lieberman, D. (2021). *Exercised: the science of physical activity, rest and health*. Penguin Books.

6 World Health Organization. (2020). *WHO guidelines on physical activity and sedentary behaviour*. World Health Organization. www.who.int/publications/i/item/9789240015128

7 Patel, A. V., Maliniak, M. L., Rees-Punia, E., Matthews, C. E., & Gapstur, S. M. (2018). Prolonged leisure time spent sitting in

relation to cause-specific mortality in a large US cohort. *American Journal of Epidemiology*, 187(10), 2151–2158. https://academic.oup.com/aje/article-abstract/187/10/2151/5045572

8 Chartered Institute of Personnel and Development (CIPD) & Simply health. (2025). *Health and wellbeing at work 2025: survey report*. CIPD. www.cipd.org/uk/knowledge/reports/health-well-being-work/

9 World Health Organization & International Labour Organization. (2021). *Long working hours increasing deaths from heart disease and stroke: WHO, ILO*, 17 May. World Health Organization. www.who.int/news/item/17-05-2021-long-working-hours-increasing-deaths-from-heart-disease-and-stroke-who-ilo. For further academic detail: Kivimäki, M., Jokela, M., Nyberg, S. T., Singh-Manoux, A., Fransson, E. I., Alfredsson, L., & The IPD-Work Consortium. (2015). Long working hours and risk of coronary heart disease and stroke: a systematic review and meta-analysis of published and unpublished data for 603,838 individuals. *The Lancet*, 386(10005), 1739–1746. www.thelancet.com/article/S0140-6736(15)60295-1/fulltext

10 Chauntry, A. J., Bishop, N. C., Hamer, M., & Paine, N. J. (2023). Frequently interrupting prolonged sitting with light body-weighted resistance activity alters psychobiological responses to acute psychological stress: a randomized crossover trial. *Annals of Behavioral Medicine*, 57(4), 301–312. https://academic.oup.com/abm/article-abstract/57/4/301/6675467

11 European Agency for Safety and Health at Work (EU-OSHA). (2022). *Get moving at work: promoting dynamic working in sedentary jobs*. Healthy Workplaces Campaign 2020–2022. Publications Office of the European Union.

12 Chartered Institute of Personnel and Development (CIPD) & Simply health. (2025). *Health and wellbeing at work 2025: survey report*. CIPD. www.cipd.org/uk/knowledge/reports/health-well-being-work/

13 Levine, J. A., Vander Weg, M. W., Hill, J. O., & Klesges, R. C. (2005). Non-exercise activity thermogenesis: The crouching tiger hidden dragon of societal weight gain. *Arteriosclerosis, Thrombosis, and Vascular Biology*, 26(4), 729–736.

14 Thompson, W. R., Arena, R., Riebe, D., Pescatello, L. S., & ACSM. (2024). 2025 ACSM worldwide fitness trends: future directions of the health and fitness industry. *ACSM's Health and Fitness Journal*, 28(6), 19–30. https://journals.lww.com/acsm-healthfitness/fulltext/2024/11000/2025_acsm_worldwide_fitness_trends__future.6.aspx

15 Michie, S., van Stralen, M. M., & West, R. (2011). The behaviour change wheel: a new method for characterising and designing behaviour change interventions. *Implementation Science*, 6(1), 42. https://doi.org/10.1186/1748-5908-6-42

16 Achor, S. (2010). *The happiness advantage: the seven principles of positive psychology that fuel success and performance at work.* Crown Business.

3 Your Nutrition Habit

1 Benton, D., Dufort, A., & Gregory, E. (2020). Healthy lifestyle behaviors: the optimal nutrition to combat burnout. In *Humanism and resilience in residency training* (pp. 371–402). Springer International Publishing.

2 The term *Mediterranean diet* was popularized by American physiologist Ancel Keys in the 1950s. Through his work on the Seven Countries Study, he observed that populations in southern Italy and Greece enjoyed notably low rates of cardiovascular disease and longer life expectancy, despite modest medical resources. Their diet, rich in vegetables, legumes, wholegrains, olive oil, and fish, was simple, seasonal, and deeply rooted in community. What stood out wasn't just *what* they ate, but *how* they ate: slowly, socially, and seasonally. At its heart, the Mediterranean approach is about balance, simplicity, and nourishment. Keys, A., & Keys, M. (1975). *How to eat well and stay well the Mediterranean way.* Doubleday. Further reading: Buettner, D. (2019). *The Blue Zones kitchen.* National Geographic.

3 Gómez-Donoso, C., Sánchez-Villegas, A., Martínez-González, M. A., Gea, A., de Deus Mendonça, R., Lahortiga-Ramos, F., & Bes-Rastrollo,

M. (2020). Ultra-processed food consumption and the incidence of depression in a Mediterranean cohort: The SUN Project. *European Journal of Nutrition*, 59(3), 1093–1103. https://doi.org/10.1007/s00394-019-01970-1

4 Philpotts, R. (2023). *The burnout bible*. Practical Inspiration.

5 Spector, T. (2015). *The diet myth: the real science behind what we eat*. Weidenfeld and Nicolson. Spector is Professor of Genetic Epidemiology at King's College London and the founder of the ZOE nutrition project. The ZOE nutrition project is a science-backed personalized nutrition programme that uses microbiome testing and continuous glucose data to help people understand how their bodies respond to food.

6 Chris van Tulleken is an infectious diseases doctor, researcher, and science communicator. His book explores how ultra-processed foods dominate modern diets, how they affect brain and body function, and why they're linked to rising rates of obesity, low mood, and poor energy regulation. Van Tulleken, C. (2023). *Ultra-processed people: why do we all eat stuff that isn't food and why can't we stop?* Cornerstone Press.

7 Adan, A. (2012). Cognitive performance and dehydration. *Journal of the American College of Nutrition*, 31(2), 71–78.

8 Walker, M. (2017). *Why we sleep: unlocking the power of sleep and dreams*. Penguin.

9 For quick and healthy meal inspiration, see Jamie Oliver (2017). *5 ingredients: quick & easy food*. Michael Joseph, or Michael Pollan (2009). *Food rules: an eater's manual*. Penguin Press.

10 James Clear is the author of *Atomic habits* (2018), a bestselling guide to behaviour change and habit formation, which draws from a range of behavioural science research. Clear, J. (2018). *Atomic habits: an easy and proven way to build good habits and break bad ones*. Avery.

11 Duhigg, C. (2012). *The power of habit: why we do what we do in life and business*. Random House.

4 Your Balance Habit

1 Deloitte. (2023). *Workplace burnout survey.* www2.deloitte.com/us/en/pages/about-deloitte/articles/burnout-survey.html
Deloitte. (2023). *Poor mental health costs UK employers £51 billion a year.* www.deloitte.com/uk/en/about/press-room/poor-mental-health-costs-uk-employers-51-billion-a-year-for-employees.html
Deloitte. (2023). *Two thirds of UK Gen Zs and millennials opt for remote and hybrid working.* www.deloitte.com/uk/en/about/press-room/two-thirds-of-uk-gen-zs-and-millennials-opt-for-remote-and-hybrid-working.html

2 For example, Deloitte's *2023 human capital trends* report highlights the growing shift away from rigid work–life boundaries, with employees across global markets expressing a desire for more personalized, flexible approaches to integrating work and life. Deloitte. (2023). *2023 global human capital trends: new fundamentals for a boundaryless world.* Deloitte Insights. www.deloitte.com/us/en/insights/topics/talent/human-capital-trends/2023.html

3 Helen Tupper and Sarah Ellis, authors of *The squiggly career* and hosts of the *Squiggly Careers* podcast, popularized the concept of 'work–life fit' in recent years, especially within the UK career and wellbeing space. The term was first used by Cali Williams Yost, a US-based workplace strategist and author of the book: Yost, C. W. (2013). *Tweak it: make what matters to you happen every day.* Center Street.

4 Adapted from Tupper, H., & Ellis, S. (2022). *You coach you: how to overcome challenges and take control of your career.* Penguin Business.

5 Psychologist Carol Dweck's pioneering work on mindset explores how developing a growth mindset supports the idea that we can adapt our habits, change how we manage energy, and recover more quickly from setbacks. Dweck, C. S. (2006). *Mindset: the new psychology of success.* Random House.

6 Tupper, H., & Ellis, S. (2022). *You coach you: how to overcome challenges and take control of your career.* Penguin Business.

7 Achor, S. (2010). *The happiness advantage: the seven principles of positive psychology that fuel success and performance at work.* Crown Business.

8 Dweck, C. S. (2006). *Mindset: the new psychology of success*. Random House.

9 The concept of the stress cycle is rooted in decades of research on the human stress response, from Walter Cannon's 'fight-or-flight' model, to Hans Selye's General Adaptation Syndrome, to Bruce McEwen's work on allostatic load. The Nagoski sisters have helped translate these physiological principles into an accessible wellbeing framework that empowers people to actively complete the stress response and prevent long-term burnout. Cannon, W. B. (1932). *The wisdom of the body*. W. W. Norton and Company. Selye, H. (1956). *The stress of life*. McGraw-Hill. McEwen, B. S. (2000). Allostasis and allostatic load: implications for neuropsychopharmacology. *Neuropsychopharmacology*, 22(2), 108–124. www.nature.com/articles/1395453. Nagoski, E., & Nagoski, A. (2019). *Burnout: the secret to unlocking the stress cycle*. Ballantine Books.

10 Christina Maslach and Michael Leiter are among the most respected researchers in the field of occupational burnout. Maslach's work helped define the term and led to the development of the Maslach Burnout Inventory, the gold standard tool used globally to measure burnout. Maslach, C., & Leiter, M. P. (1997). *The truth about burnout: how organizations cause personal stress and what to do about it*. Jossey-Bass.

11 For more on how flexible and hybrid working are reshaping expectations of work–life integration, see: Chartered Institute of Personnel and Development. (2023). *Flexible working: the business case*. CIPD. www.cipd.org/globalassets/media/knowledge/knowledge-hub/reports/2023-pdfs/2023-flexible-working-the-business-case-august.pdf

12 McKinsey Health Institute. (2023). *Addressing employee burnout: are you solving the right problem?* www.mckinsey.com/mhi/our-insights/addressing-employee-burnout-are-you-solving-the-right-problem

13 Wood, W. (2019). *Good habits, bad habits: the science of making positive changes that stick*. Macmillan Business.

5 Your Rest Habit

1 Niazi, A., Memon, M. A., Sarwar, N., Obaid, A., Mirza, M. Z., & Amjad, K. (2024). Work intensification: a systematic review of studies from 1989–2022. *Work*, 77(3), 769–787. https://pubmed.ncbi.nlm.nih.gov/37781853/

2 Microsoft. (2025). *Breaking down the infinite workday* (Work Trend Index Annual Report). Microsoft. www.microsoft.com/en-us/worklab/work-trend-index/breaking-down-infinite-workday

3 Gallup. (2022). *State of the global workplace: 2022 report*. www.gallup.com/workplace/349484/state-of-the-global-workplace-2022-report.aspx

4 Hammond, C. (2019). *The art of rest: how to find respite in the modern age*. Canongate Books.

5 Leroy, S. (2009). Why is it so hard to do my work? The challenge of attention residue when switching between work tasks. *Organizational Behavior and Human Decision Processes*, 109(2), 168–181. www.sciencedirect.com/science/article/abs/pii/S0749597809000399

6 Huberman, A. D. (2023, February 5). *Breathwork protocols for health, focus & stress*. Huberman Lab. www.hubermanlab.com/newsletter/breathwork-protocols-for-health-focus-stress

7 Jha, A. P. (2021). *Peak mind: find your focus, own your attention, invest 12 minutes a day*. Harper Wave.

8 Chatterjee, R. (2018). *The stress solution: the 4 steps to reset your body, mind, relationships and purpose*. Penguin Life.

9 Newport, C. (2016). *Deep work: rules for focused success in a distracted world*. Grand Central Publishing.

10 Saundra Dalton-Smith is an internal medicine physician and wellbeing researcher whose book *Sacred rest* draws on clinical experience and scientific evidence to reveal how different types of rest impact health and performance. Dalton-Smith, S. (2017). *Sacred rest: recover your life, renew your energy, restore your sanity*. Faith Words.

11 Siegel, D. J. (2012). *The whole-brain child: 12 revolutionary strategies to nurture your child's developing mind*. Scribe Publications.

12 To explore the science of mindfulness further, see the work of Jon Kabat-Zinn, creator of the Mindfulness-Based Stress Reduction programme. Kabat-Zinn, J. (2013). *Full catastrophe living: using the wisdom of your body and mind to face stress, pain, and illness* (revised ed.). Bantam Books.

13 Søberg, S. (2022). *Winter swimming: the Nordic way towards a healthier and happier life*. Quercus (MacLehose Press).

14 Gielan, M. (2015). *Broadcasting happiness: the science of igniting and sustaining positive change*. BenBella Books.

15 For more information on recognizing and managing perimenopause symptoms, see NICE Guidelines on Menopause or visit www.nhs.uk/conditions/menopause/

16 Clear, J. (2018). *Atomic habits: an easy and proven way to build good habits and break bad ones*. Avery.

17 Sir Dave Brailsford's 'marginal gains' philosophy is explored by Matthew Syed (2015). *Black box thinking: the surprising truth about success*. John Murray. And referenced in *Atomic habits* by James Clear (2018), where it's linked to sustainable habit change and peak performance. Clear, J. (2018). *Atomic habits: an easy and proven way to build good habits and break bad ones*. Avery.

6 Your Connection Habit

1 In Murthy's book *Together*, he describes loneliness as a public health crisis with wide-reaching implications for emotional and physical wellbeing. He advocates for reimagining workplaces and communities to prioritize connection, not just as a personal choice, but as a cultural and organizational priority. Murthy, V. H. (2020). *Together: the healing power of human connection in a sometimes lonely world*. Harper Wave.

2 Holt-Lunstad, J., Robles, T. F., & Sbarra, D. A. (2017). Advancing social connection as a public health priority in the United States. *American Psychologist*, 72(6), 517–530. https://doi.org/10.1037%2Famp0000103

3 Holt-Lunstad, J., Smith, T. B., & Layton, J. B. (2010). Social relationships and mortality risk: a meta-analytic review. *PLOS Medicine*, 7(7), e1000316. https://doi.org/10.1371/journal.pmed.1000316. This landmark study analysed data from over 300,000 people and found that strong social relationships increase the odds of survival by 50%. The health risk of chronic loneliness was shown to be a critical, yet often overlooked factor in physical health and longevity.

4 Dunbar, R. (2021). *Friends: understanding the power of our most important relationships*. Little, Brown Spark.

5 Murthy, V. H. (2020). *Together: the healing power of human connection in a sometimes lonely world*. Harper Wave.

6 The Harvard Study of Adult Development is one of the longest-running longitudinal studies in psychology. Directed by psychiatrist Robert Waldinger, you can find out more about the study in his book *The Good Life*. Waldinger, R. J., & Schulz, M. S. (2023). *The good life: lessons from the world's longest scientific study of happiness*. Simon and Schuster.

7 Van Lange, P. A. M. (2020). Social connection as a basic human need: the need to belong and the need to trust. In R. J. Sternberg & S. T. Fiske (Eds.), *The Cambridge handbook of wisdom* (pp. 367–381). Cambridge University Press.

8 Carter, C. S. (2014). Oxytocin pathways and the evolution of human behavior. *Annual Review of Psychology*, 65, 17–39. https://doi.org/10.1146/annurev-psych-010213-115110

9 Fredrickson, B. L., & Losada, M. F. (2005). Positive affect and the complex dynamics of human flourishing. *American Psychologist*, 60(7), 678–686. https://doi.org/10.1037%2F0003-066X.60.7.678 The mathematical model used by Losada was later critiqued for being overly simplified. That said, the core finding that more positive interactions create healthier team dynamics is well supported across fields like positive psychology and organizational behaviour.

10 John Gottman's 'Love Lab' at the University of Washington observed thousands of couples to identify communication patterns that predict long-term success or breakdown. His 5:1 ratio became one of

his most widely referenced findings in relationship psychology and is now often used in team development and leadership coaching as a model for building trust and resilience. Gottman, J. M., & Silver, N. (2015). *The seven principles for making marriage work: a practical guide from the country's foremost relationship expert*. Harmony.

11 Gallup. (2023). *State of the global workplace 2023 report*. Gallup, Inc. www.gallup.com/workplace/349484/state-of-the-global-workplace.aspx

12 McKinsey and Company research by Alexander, A., Cracknell, R., De Smet, A., Langstaff, M., & Ravid, D. (2022). *The state of hybrid work: making it fit with your strategy*. McKinsey and Company. Also Gallup. (2023). *State of the global workplace 2023 report*. Gallup, Inc. www.gallup.com/workplace/349484/state-of-the-global-workplace.aspx

13 Achor, S. (2013). *Before happiness: the 5 hidden keys to achieving success, spreading happiness, and sustaining positive change*. Crown Business.

14 Gielan, M. (2015). *Broadcasting happiness: the science of igniting and sustaining positive change*. BenBella Books.

15 Insights discussed at length in my *Wellbeing Trailblazers* group but the philosophy is attributed to author Derek Sivers. Sivers, D. (2011). *Anything you want: 40 lessons for a new kind of entrepreneur*. Penguin Books.

16 Hormonal fluctuations particularly during menstrual, perimenopausal, and menopausal phases can influence mood, emotional sensitivity, and energy regulation. For more, see Brizendine, L. (2022). *The upgrade: how the female brain gets stronger and better in midlife and beyond*. Harmony Books. Also, Sims, S., & Yeager, S. (2022). *Next level: your guide to kicking ass, feeling great, and crushing goals through menopause and beyond*. Rodale Books.

17 Rangan Chatterjee, in his book *The Stress Solution* (2018), champions *nature prescriptions*, recommending even 10–20 minutes outdoors as a daily wellbeing habit for reducing overwhelm and boosting mental clarity. Chatterjee, R. (2018). *The stress solution: the 4 steps to a calmer, happier, healthier you*. Penguin Life.

18 Chatterjee, R. (2022). *Happy mind, happy life: 10 simple ways to feel great every day*. Penguin Life.

19 Beetz, A., Uvnäs-Moberg, K., Julius, H., & Kotrschal, K. (2012). Psychosocial and psychophysiological effects of human-animal interactions: the possible role of oxytocin. *Frontiers in Psychology*, 3, 234. https://doi.org/10.3389/fpsyg.2012.00234

20 Although data created by wearables is anonymized, privacy can be a concern. A transparent data policy is paramount, as is making it clear what the benefits to the employee will be.

21 Milkman, K. (2021). *How to change: the science of getting from where you are to where you want to be*. Penguin Random House.

22 Graham, E. K., Beck, E. D., Jackson, K., Yoneda, T., McGhee, C., Pieramici, L., Atherton, O. E., Luo, J., Willroth, E. C., Steptoe, A., Mroczek, D. K., & Ong, A. D. (2024). Do we become more lonely with age? A coordinated data analysis of nine longitudinal studies. *Psychological Science*, 35(6), 579–596. https://pubmed.ncbi.nlm.nih.gov/38687352/

7 Your Sleep Habit

1 The Sleep School. (2021). *National sleep survey*. Dr Guy Meadows and The Sleep School. www.thesleepschool.org

2 For more on global sleep health, visit the World Sleep Society, an international organization supporting evidence-based education and awareness across over 80 countries. These align with UK guidelines available from: National Health Service (NHS). (2023). *How to fall asleep faster and sleep better.* www.nhs.uk/every-mind-matters/mental-wellbeing-tips/how-to-fall-asleep-faster-and-sleep-better/

3 Walker, M. (2017). *Why we sleep: unlocking the power of sleep and dreams*. Scribner.

4 Syed, M. (2015). *Black box thinking: the surprising truth about success*. John Murray.

5 Mah, C. D., Mah, K. E., Kezirian, E. J., & Dement, W. C. (2011). The effects of sleep extension on the athletic performance of collegiate basketball players. *Sleep*, 34(7), 943–950. For comprehensive and up-to-date information on sleep and athletic performance, check out this expert consensus paper: Walsh, N. P., Halson, S. L., Sargent, C., et al. (2021). Sleep and the athlete: narrative review and 2021 expert consensus recommendations. *British Journal of Sports Medicine*, 55(7), 356–368. www.sportgeneeskunde.com/wp-content/uploads/Br-J-Sports-Med-2021-Walsh-consensus-statement-sleep-and-the-athlete.pdf

6 Littlehales, N. (2016). *Sleep: the myth of 8 hours, the power of naps… and the new plan to recharge your body and mind.* Penguin Life.

7 Roenneberg, T. (2012). *Internal time: chronotypes, social jet lag, and why you're so tired.* Harvard University Press.

8 Walker, M. (2017). *Why we sleep: unlocking the power of sleep and dreams.* Scribner.

9 Breus, M. J. (2016). *The power of when: discover your chronotype and the best time to eat lunch, ask for a raise, have sex, write a novel, take your meds, and more.* Little, Brown Spark.

10 To discover your chronotype and explore personalized energy strategies, take Michael Breus's free quiz at www.thepowerofwhenquiz.com

11 A cognitive neuroscientist and professor at UC Irvine, Mednick is known for her work on sleep architecture and naps. Mednick, S. C., & Ehrman, M. (2006). *Take a nap! Change your life: the scientific plan to make you smarter, healthier, more productive.* Workman Publishing.

12 Lembke, A. (2021). *Dopamine nation: finding balance in the age of indulgence.* Dutton.

13 Walker, M. (2017). *Why we sleep: unlocking the power of sleep and dreams.* Scribner.

14 Chang, A.-M., Aeschbach, D., Duffy, J. F., & Czeisler, C. A. (2015). Evening use of light-emitting eReaders negatively affects sleep,

circadian timing, and next-morning alertness. *Proceedings of the National Academy of Sciences*, 112(4), 1232–1237. https://doi.org/10.1073/pnas.1418490112

15 Walker, M. (2017). *Why we sleep: the new science of sleep and dreams*. Penguin Books.

16 Clear, J. (2018). *Atomic habits: an easy & proven way to build good habits & break bad ones*. Avery.

Index

A quick word from Practical Inspiration Publishing...

We hope you found this book both practical and inspiring – that's what we aim for with every book we publish.

We publish titles on topics ranging from leadership, entrepreneurship, HR and marketing to self-development and wellbeing.

Find details of all our books at: www.practicalinspiration.com

Did you know...

We can offer discounts on bulk sales of all our titles – ideal if you want to use them for training purposes, corporate giveaways or simply because you feel these ideas deserve to be shared with your network.

We can even produce bespoke versions of our books, for example with your organization's logo and/or a tailored foreword.

To discuss further, contact us on info@practicalinspiration.com.

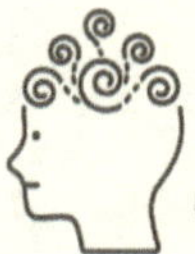

Got an idea for a business book?

We may be able to help. Find out about more about publishing in partnership with us at: bit.ly/PIpublishing.

Follow us on social media...

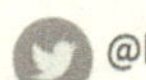 @PIPTalking

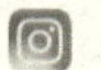 @pip_talking

 @practicalinspiration

 @piptalking

 Practical Inspiration Publishing

www.ingramcontent.com/pod-product-compliance
Lightning Source LLC
LaVergne TN
LVHW050955080826
845145LV00006B/1509

* 9 7 8 1 7 8 8 6 0 8 8 5 5 *